The Companion Exercise Forms for

Teach Me Language

A language manual for children with autism, Asperger's syndrome and related developmental disorders.

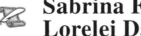 Sabrina Freeman Ph.D.
Lorelei Dake B.A.

Copyright © 1997 by SKF Books. All rights reserved.

No part of this book may be reproduced in any form or by any means without the prior written permission of the publisher, with the exception of pages designated for use in language programs. These pages may be reproduced by parents for use with their own child, or by professionals for use with their clients, but not for distribution to a group of professionals or parents, a school district, school, or clinic.

The Companion Exercise Forms For Teach Me Language (known as the Companion Exercise Forms), is intended only for use with *Teach Me Language: A Language Manual for Children with Autism, Asperger's Syndrome and Related Developmental Disorders*. The Companion Exercise Forms must only be used in conjunction with the *Teach Me Language* manual which contains detailed instructions on the use of the Companion Exercise Forms.

Although *Teach Me Language* and the *Companion Exercise Forms* are intended for parents of children with autism, Asperger's syndrome or related developmental disorders, the authors and publisher must emphasize that the exercises in this book are a guide to be used as part of a therapy program overseen by professional consultants, and should not be used without the professional guidance of either a behavioral consultant or speech pathologist. Both *Teach Me Language* and the *Companion Exercise Forms* are not a substitute for a professionally designed language education program.

Any errors and omissions are the responsibility of the first author, Dr. Sabrina Freeman.

Library of Congress Cataloging-in-Publication Data

Freeman, Sabrina
Teach me language

Includes index.
1. Autistic children--Education--Language arts.
2. Developmentally disabled children--Education--Language arts.
I. Dake, Lorelei II. Title.
LC4717.U43 1997 Supplement   371.92'8046   C96-910537-1

SKF Books,
20641 46th Avenue,
Langley, B.C.
CANADA V3A 3H8

ISBN: 0-9657565-1-3
Printed in the United States of America
First Edition

Contents

Chapter 1: Introduction
Why These Forms Need the Teach Me Language Manual 8
Why We Wrote the Companion Forms for Teach Me Language 8
Use of the Exercise Sheets 9
Understanding How to Do the Exercises 9
Customizing the Exercise Sheets 9

Chapter 2: Social Language Companion Forms
Simple Word Associations 12
Contingent Word Work Sheet 13
Building Analogies (Identifying Word Relationships) 14
Pretend Play Work Sheet 15
Topical Conversation Activity Sheet (1) 16
Topical Conversation Activity Sheet (2) 17
Conversation Record 18
Finding Out About Someone (1) 19
Finding Out About Someone (2) 20
Finding Out About Someone (3) 21
Finding Out About Someone (4) 22
Making Comments and Asking Questions 23
Topical Questions/Comments For Conversation 24
Conversational Self-Monitoring 25
Emotions Sheet 26
Determining A Cause 27
Identifying Situations: Emotions/ Consequences 28
Problems, People's Reactions & Solutions 29
Identifying If A Situation is Safe or Dangerous 30
Identifying If There is a Problem 31
Deciding What To Do 32
Problem/Solutions 33
Identifying "Trouble" and Generating Solutions 34
Identifying If Someone is Being Made Fun Of 35
Identifying If Something Said is Nice Or Mean 36
Multiple Opinions 37
Opinions and Supporting Reasons: Food 38
Opinions and Supporting Reasons: Movies 39
Fact Or Opinion? 40
My Opinions (About School) 41
My Opinions (About Movies) 42

Chapter 3: General Knowledge Companion Forms
Outline For Topical Information 44
Simple Child - Generated Outline 45
Simple Outline with Elaborative Statement 46
Multi-Paragraph Outline 47
Oral Definitions: Animals 48
Animal Grid Fill-In (Introduction to Animal Comparisons) 49
True or False? (1) 50
True or False? (2) 51
Outline For Topical Information 52
Simple Child - Generated Outline 53
Simple Outline with Elaborative Statement 54
Multi-Paragraph Outline 55
Multi-Paragraph Outline 55
Oral Definitions: Occupations 56
Occupation Grid Fill-In (Introduction to Occupation Comparisons) 57
Who Would Say This? 58

What Would They Say? 59
Current Topics 60
Making Comparisons 61
Grid Comparison (Animal, Occupation Sport, etc...) 62
+/- Comparison (Animal, Occupation, Sport, etc...) 63
Sport Comparisons Using "Both" 64
General Comparisons (1) 65
General Comparisons (2) 66

Chapter 4: Grammar and Syntax Companion Forms

Classifying Pronouns 68
Pronoun Referents Exercise 69
Super Sentences 70
Identifying Phrases 71

Chapter 5: Advanced Language Development Companion Forms

Easy Story Writing 74
Intermediate Story Writing 75
Difficult Story Writing 76
Advanced Story Writing 77
Easy Story Pre-Writing 78
Difficult Story Pre-Writing 79
Advanced Story Pre-writing 80
Writing a Topic Sentence 81
Outline for Paragraph Writing & Topical Conversation - Easy 82
Outline for Paragraph Writing and Topical 83
Conversation - Intermediate 83
Outline for Paragraph Writing and Topical Conversation - Advanced 84
Writing a Paragraph 85
Developing Your Story (Introductory Paragraph) 86
Developing Your Story - Paragraph 2 87
Developing Your Story - Paragraph 3 88
Developing Your Story - Paragraph 4 89
Finding the Main Idea 90
Sentence Starters For Descriptive Topic Sentences and Detail Sentences of Support 91
Two-Column Notes 92
Letter Template 93
What I Did Today: (What Did You Do Today?) 94
Daily Routine Sheet (Recall of Day) 95

Chapter 6: Academic/Language Based Concept Companion Forms

Simple Categorization: Nouns 98
Simple Categorization: Verbs 99
Simple Categorization: Naming Items 100
Familiar Words: Identifying the Group & Function 101
Object Functions: Fill-Ins 102
Categorization 103
Brainstorming 104
Pre-Reading Comprehension: 105
Who? and What did (or do)? 105
Pre-Reading Comprehension: 106
Who? and What did (or do)? 106
Important Story Events 107
Story Sequence 108
Story Report 109
Story Summary 110
Summarizing Independently 111
Reading Comprehension Record 112
Identifying the Kind of Text Read 113
Event or Detail? 114

Math Word Problems 115
New Vocabulary 116
Orally Defining Words (Objects) 117
Orally Defining Words (People) 118
Orally Defining Words (Verbs) 119
Vocabulary and Synonyms - Easy 120
Using New Vocabulary: Stories 121
Applying New Vocabulary 122
New Vocabulary for the Week 123
New Vocabulary To Be Reinforced 124
Ordering Information 125
Sequencing and Ordering 126
Comparing Numbers 127
Understanding Place Value 128
Using Comparatives - Sheet 1 129
Using Comparatives - Sheet 2 130
Monthly Calendar Fill-In 131
Using The Correct Verb Tense 132
What Happens? 133
AM Or PM Time 134
Sequencing Time 135
Comparing Time 136
Time Equivalents 137
Time Questions 138
When Phrases 139
Comparing Money - Sheet 1 140
Comparing Money - Sheet 2 141
Sequencing And Ordering 142
Do I Have Enough Money? - Sheet 1 143
Do I Have Enough Money - Sheet 2 144
Buying Things & Working With Money 145
Money Questions (Auditory) 146
Agents and Their Actions 147
Verbal Analogies 148

Chapter 7: Therapy Schedule Companion Forms
Simplified Schedule For The Child 150
Independent Work Instrument 151
Weekly Drill/Activity Record 152

1 Introduction
Forms

- Why These Forms Need the Teach Me Language Manual
- Why We Wrote the Companion Forms for Teach Me Language
- Use of the Exercise Sheets
- Understanding How to Do the Exercises
- Customizing the Exercise Sheets

Introduction

Why These Forms Need the *Teach Me Language* Manual

Before using the *Companion Exercise Forms for Teach Me Language*, it is very important to read and understand the "How To" and "Why" sections in the *Teach Me Language* manual. When working with children with autism spectrum disorders, the material must be taught in a way that sets the child up for success. Without understanding how to introduce the various exercises, the child can become frustrated and "turn off" learning. The instructions which accompany each exercise in the *Teach Me Language* manual are also important to help you decide if the child is ready for the exercise.

Why We Wrote the *Companion Forms for Teach Me Language*

The *Companion Exercise Forms for Teach Me Language* makes the *Teach Me Language* manual more convenient to use because it provides all the manual's exercise forms in a larger, blank format. To help explain how the exercises in *Teach Me Language* are done, the book includes facsimiles of drill sheets, filled out with examples of how and why the exercises are done. A sample is illustrated below.

The *Teach Me Language* manual - sample pages

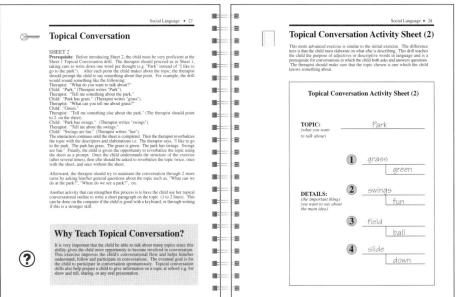

The *Companion Exercise Forms for Teach Me Language* is a collection of the exercise sheets found in the *Teach Me Language* manual without the examples written on the forms. The exercise forms in this supplement are blank and enlarged for ease of use.

EXERCISE/DRILL

All the pages in the *Teach Me Language* manual where the exercise/drill symbol appears, are included in this supplement without examples of how to do the drills. Examples of completed exercise forms, and instructions in their use, are in the *Teach Me Language* manual.

Use of the Exercise Sheets

The exercise forms in this supplement are designed to be photocopied and used in the child's program. The ability to make several copies is important because the exercises need to be done several times, gradually increasing the level of ability as the child learns the material. It is a good idea to photocopy the forms rather than use the originals in this supplement so a complete set of blank originals is always on hand.

Understanding How to Do the Exercises

In order to do the exercises in this supplement effectively, it is important to know that they are not self explanatory for the child. They must be introduced to the child by the adult who presents each part of the exercise and demonstrates correct sample answers. To complete the exercise independently (where indicated), the child should be very familiar with the exercise. This may require doing the exercise many times with an adult. To achieve this method of teaching, the adult must be very familiar with the exercise before working on it with the child. This is why this book of companion forms cannot stand alone. The *Teach Me Language* manual is needed to know how the exercises are done effectively.

Customizing the Exercise Sheets

The exercise sheets have been designed to be as easy to use as possible for the child; however, if required, they can be tailored to each child's program to make them more effective. Some of the exercises can also be done on a dry-erase board. Some children find it motivating to write on and erase a board.

2 Social Language
Forms

- Simple Word Associations
- Contingent Word Work Sheet
- Building Analogies (Identifying Word Relationships)
- Pretend Play Work Sheet
- Topical Conversation Activity Sheet (1)
- Topical Conversation Activity Sheet (2)
- Conversation Record
- Finding Out About Someone (1)
- Finding Out About Someone (2)
- Finding Out About Someone (3)
- Finding Out About Someone (4)
- Making Comments and Asking Questions
- Topical Questions/Comments For Conversation
- Conversational Self-Monitoring
- Emotions Sheet
- Determining a Cause
- Identifying Situations: Emotions/Consequences
- Problems, People's Reactions & Solutions
- Identifying If A Situation is Safe or Dangerous
- Identifying If There is a Problem
- Deciding What To Do
- Problem/Solutions
- Identifying "Trouble" and Generating Solutions
- Identifying If Someone is Being Made Fun Of
- Identifying If Something Said is Nice Or Mean
- Multiple Opinions
- Opinions and Supporting Reasons: Food
- Opinions and Supporting Reasons: Movies
- Fact or Opinion?
- My Opinions (About School)
- My Opinions (About Movies)

Forms in this chapter accompany Teach Me Language. Complete instructions on their use are in Chapter 2 of Teach Me Language. Copyright © 1997 SKF Books.

# Simple Word Associations

Word   Paired Word   Reason

_____   _____

_____   _____

_____   _____

_____   _____

_____   _____

Simple Word Associations The simple word association exercise can be done in two ways. The way to introduce this drill is to have the therapist write down a word pair and ask the child why the two words go together. The second way to do this drill is to have the child give a word that relates to the one word the therapist suggests. Then the child must "explain" why s/he chose the word (e.g. why s/he chose flower to go with butterfly). Once the child can do this with relative ease, s/he can move on to "The Contingent Word" exercise.

This form accompanies *Teach Me Language*. Complete instructions on its use are in Chapter 2 of *Teach Me Language*.
Copyright © 1997 SKF Books.

Contingent Word Work Sheet

_____ – _____ – _____ – _____ – _____

_____ – _____ – _____ – _____ – _____

_____ – _____ – _____ – _____ – _____

_____ – _____ – _____ – _____ – _____

_____ – _____ – _____ – _____ – _____

Contingent Word Work Sheet This exercise structures a conversation of sorts, since the child is able to share his/her thoughts without putting them into a sentence. There is turn taking where the child and the therapist both must concentrate on what the other is saying, since the next word must relate to the preceding word. Once the sheet is completed, the child can choose one of the lines and explain why the two words go together. This exercise is one of the easiest exercises with which to start the social language chapter.

This form accompanies Teach Me Language. Complete instructions on its use are in Chapter 2 of Teach Me Language.
Copyright © 1997 SKF Books.

Building Analogies (Identifying Word Relationships)

In each box an arrow is drawn from one word to another. On the line below, tell how or why the words go together (write a relationship sentence). Then find 2 other words that go together in the same way. Write the relationship sentence for the 2 words you choose. Then think of 2 more words that could go together in the same way and write your own relationship sentence.

```
┌─────────────────────────────────────────────────────────────┐
│                    Contingent Words                         │
│                                                             │
│         _____              _____                  │
│                                                             │
│   _____                              _____        │
│                                                             │
│                                                             │
│         _____              _____                  │
└─────────────────────────────────────────────────────────────┘
```

Relationship Sentence: _____

_____

Relationship Sentence: _____

_____

Two (2) more words that go together in the same way: _____

Relationship Sentence: _____

_____

Building Analogies (Identifying Word Relationships) This exercise builds the child's critical thinking skills. The therapist should do several word pairs before having the child come up with these words on his/her own. In addition, the therapist should go through a completed sheet with the child before requiring the child to do this on his/her own. Once the child understands the relationship that the therapist would like him/her to create, then the child should try the sheet on his own coming up with different relationship sentences.

This form accompanies *Teach Me Language*. Complete instructions on its use are in Chapter 2 of *Teach Me Language*. Copyright © 1997 SKF Books.

Pretend Play Work Sheet

        Item   Response   Demonstrates Play

1. _____ _____ _____

2. _____ _____ _____

3. _____ _____ _____

4. _____ _____ _____

5. _____ _____ _____

Pretend Play Work Sheet Pretend play is one of the deficits typical in children with various pervasive developmental disorders. Yet, it is an important social skill since much play involves pretending amongst younger children. This activity structures pretend play in its simplest form. Once the child understands the exercise, it is a good idea to begin very simple pretend exercises with dolls e.g. the child can be taught to pretend that the doll is swimming, eating or going to sleep. Once the child understands pretend play with dolls, then the next step is to create a very simple story about a doll going to do an activity. Once the child can tell a story about a doll, the therapist can create scripts to act out using dolls. Some children will take these skills and generalize them in their free time. This work sheet is for the therapist and should not be used by the child.

This form accompanies Teach Me Language. Complete instructions on its use are in Chapter 2 of Teach Me Language.
Copyright © 1997 SKF Books.

Topical Conversation Activity Sheet (1)

TOPIC: _____
*(what you want
to talk about)*

① _____

DETAILS: ② _____
*(the important things
you want to say about
the main idea)*

③ _____

④ _____

Topical Conversation Activity Sheet (1) This exercise teaches the child the basic structure of a conversation in which the child must describe a topic and answer questions on that topic. This is a prerequisite for conversations in which the child both asks and answers questions. The therapist should make sure the topic chosen is one which the child knows something about.

This form accompanies *Teach Me Language*. Complete instructions on its use are in Chapter 2 of *Teach Me Language*.
Copyright © 1997 SKF Books.

Topical Conversation Activity Sheet (2)

TOPIC: _____
*(what you want
to talk about)*

① _____
   _____

DETAILS:
*(the important things
you want to say about
the main idea)*

② _____
   _____

③ _____
   _____

④ _____
   _____

Topical Conversation Activity Sheet (2) This more advanced exercise is similar to the initial exercise. The difference here is that the child must elaborate on what s/he is describing. This drill teaches the child the purpose of adjectives or descriptive words in language and is a prerequisite for conversations in which the child both asks and answers questions. The therapist should make sure that the topic chosen is one which the child knows something about.

This form accompanies Teach Me Language. Complete instructions on its use are in Chapter 2 of Teach Me Language.
Copyright © 1997 SKF Books.

Conversation Record

Date: _____   Where: _____

                                    Who   What

☐ Ask a question; _____   _____
   Say/ask 2   _____
   more things   _____

☐ Ask a question; _____   _____
   Say/ask 2   _____
   more things   _____

☐ Ask a question; _____   _____
   Say/ask 2   _____
   more things   _____

Conversation Record The child should have a Conversation Record taped to his/her desk everyday at school and at home during therapy. If this is done consistently, the child will be engaged in conversation 6 times per day. At first, the child will need considerable prompting until s/he realizes that s/he is accountable for initiating and recording some sort of conversation 3 times per setting. The child must learn to fill in the form (with heavy prompting at first, if necessary). After the child knows how to complete the form independently, a reinforcement/consequence system must be built in to motivate the child to complete the form.

This form accompanies *Teach Me Language*. Complete instructions on its use are in Chapter 2 of *Teach Me Language*.
Copyright © 1997 SKF Books.

Finding Out About Someone (1)

Ask _____ questions about what s/he likes.

1. __eat_____   _____

2. __drink_____   _____

3. __do_____   _____

4. __play with_____   _____

5. __go_____   _____

Finding Out About Someone This exercise is designed to give the child the necessary tools to find out about another person. The first sheet includes basic questions. The child should use the sheet to ask people these questions. Once the child has mastered these questions, the next sheet should be introduced and sheet (1) should be used periodically to maintain the questions. Eventually, the sheet should be faded out and the child should be able to ask people questions from memory.

This form accompanies Teach Me Language. Complete instructions on its use are in Chapter 2 of Teach Me Language.
Copyright © 1997 SKF Books.

Social Language • 20

Finding Out About Someone (2)

Ask _____ questions about what s/he likes.

1. __movie_____   _____

2. __book_____   _____

3. __animal_____   _____

4. __color_____   _____

5. __friend_____   _____

Finding Out About Someone (2) This exercise is designed to give the child the necessary tools to find out about another person. This second sheet includes questions that are slightly more advanced than the first. As in the first sheet, the child should use this sheet to ask people these questions. Once the child has mastered these questions, the third sheet should be introduced and this sheet (2) should be used periodically to maintain the questions. Eventually, the sheet should be faded out and the child should be able to ask people questions from memory.

This form accompanies *Teach Me Language*. Complete instructions on its use are in Chapter 2 of *Teach Me Language*.
Copyright © 1997 SKF Books.

Finding Out About Someone (3)

Ask _____ questions about what s/he likes.

1. __old/birthday__   _____

2. __live__   _____

3. __family__   _____

4. __brothers/sisters__   _____

5. __pet__   _____

Finding Out About Someone (3) This exercise is designed to give the child the necessary tools to find out about another person. This third sheet includes questions that are slightly more advanced than questions on the first and second sheets. As in the previous sheets, the child should use this sheet to ask people these questions. Once the child has mastered these questions, then the therapist and the child should use the fourth sheet to think of some questions that are truly interesting to the child. Eventually, all the sheets should be faded out and the child should be able to ask people questions from memory.

This form accompanies Teach Me Language. Complete instructions on its use are in Chapter 2 of Teach Me Language.
Copyright © 1997 SKF Books.

Social Language • 22

Finding Out About Someone (4)

Ask _____ questions about what s/he likes.

1. _____   _____

2. _____   _____

3. _____   _____

4. _____   _____

5. _____   _____

Finding Out About Someone (4) This exercise is designed to give the child the necessary tools to find out about another person. This fourth sheet includes questions the child cares about. These questions should be of genuine interest to the child. Eventually, all the sheets should be faded out and the child should be able to ask people questions from memory. *NOTE: They can ask questions they have learned from the first three sheets but not in the same order. It is good if they can come up with new questions; however, that is an advanced skill.*

This form accompanies *Teach Me Language*. Complete instructions on its use are in Chapter 2 of *Teach Me Language*.
Copyright © 1997 SKF Books.

Making Comments and Asking Questions

1. (   )   _____, what do you like to _____?
   I like _____ ↗

2. (   )   _____, what do you like to _____?
   I like _____ ↗

3. (   )   _____, what do you like to _____?
   I like _____ ↗

4. (   )   _____, what do you like to _____?
   I like _____ ↗

Making Comments and Asking Questions Once the child is good at doing the contingent word exercise, it is time to introduce contingent statements. Making comments and asking questions are basic contingent statements introduced in this drill. The child must use the verb in the parenthesis to make a comment. Then the therapist must write the question she is going to ask the child and then ask the child (e.g. "John, what do you like to eat?"). Then the child must answer the therapist. Once the child understands the relationship between the verb and the question, the child can ask the therapist a question based on the therapist's question. This introductory drill is visual, so the child can grasp the structure of the comment and question.

This form accompanies Teach Me Language. Complete instructions on its use are in Chapter 2 of Teach Me Language.
Copyright © 1997 SKF Books.

Topical Questions/Comments For Conversation

Topic: _____

Questions I can ask: Comments I can make:

_____   _____

_____   _____

_____   _____

_____   _____

Actual Conversation: (Rehearse above in Question - Response format with the therapist asking the question., Then talk about the beach without a visual prompt, and record below).

_____

_____

_____

_____

Topical Questions/Comments For Conversation This exercise structures a conversation using Who, What, Where, and Which questions. The child's responses must be written down because it should help him/her stay on task and see how the questions and responses relate to the topic. Questions that simply require a Yes or No answer should be avoided unless the child is going to expand a Yes or No answer. The therapist should NOT require the child to answer a yes or no question in a full sentence **every time** because the child will sound stilted. The actual conversation that takes place should be written down as it is happening, so 1) the child can see the conversation after it has taken place, and 2) the therapist has a record of comparison for future progress checks.

This form accompanies *Teach Me Language*. Complete instructions on its use are in Chapter 2 of *Teach Me Language*.
Copyright © 1997 SKF Books.

Social Language • 25

Conversational Self-Monitoring

My job: Keep the conversation going through at least 8 turns by asking questions and making comments.

TOPIC: _____ ☐ ☐ ☐ ☐ **?**
                                  ☐ ☐ ☐ ☐ **C**

Summary of Conversation: _____

_____

_____

TOPIC: _____ ☐ ☐ ☐ ☐ **?**
                                  ☐ ☐ ☐ ☐ **C**

Summary of Conversation: _____

_____

_____

? = question
C = comment

Conversational Self-Monitoring This form is designed to have the child monitor his/her own conversation. First, the child chooses a topic. S/he begins with either a question or a comment, and then asks a question. The therapist then answers the question. The child must either make a comment or ask a question to keep the conversation going. Every time the child makes a new statement (question or comment - question) s/he puts an X in the box. The child must keep the conversation going for at least 8 exchanges. The child uses the top row if s/he asks a question, and the second row if s/he makes a comment.

This form accompanies Teach Me Language. Complete instructions on its use are in Chapter 2 of Teach Me Language.
Copyright © 1997 SKF Books.

Emotions Sheet

Things that make me
MAD

Things that make me
HAPPY

Things that make me
SAD

I get mad when...

I am happy when...

I am sad when...

_____

_____

_____

_____

_____

_____

_____

_____

_____

_____

_____

_____

_____

_____

_____

_____

_____

_____

Emotions Sheet Before introducing any of the "Emotion, Cause and Effect" exercises, the mother, father or therapist should complete this sheet. Then the child should listen to the person read one of the emotion columns. It is a good idea to work on happy first. After a few sessions, the next emotion should be chosen. The child is simply being introduced to the emotions and will probably not gain a full understanding from this sheet; however, the sheet should be used to create the following exercises. Through those exercises the child will begin to gain an idea of how we label feelings.

This form accompanies *Teach Me Language*. Complete instructions on its use are in Chapter 2 of *Teach Me Language*.
Copyright © 1997 SKF Books.

Determining A Cause

Event/Situation　　　　　　　　　　　Cause/Why? How?

_____　　　_____

　　　　　　　　　　　　　　　　　　_____

　　　　　　　　　　　　　　　　　　_____

_____　　　_____

　　　　　　　　　　　　　　　　　　_____

_____　　　_____

　　　　　　　　　　　　　　　　　　_____

Determining A Cause This is the first exercise that makes explicit the relationship between events that the child causes and the emotional reactions to those events. It is very difficult to take these explicit relationships and have the child internalize them; however, it is important that the child have some sense that s/he can cause or avoid situations which create undesired emotions e.g. anger or sadness. This sheet must be customized to the child to make it relevant.

This form accompanies Teach Me Language. Complete instructions on its use are in Chapter 2 of Teach Me Language.
Copyright © 1997 SKF Books.

Social Language • 28

Identifying Situations: Emotions/ Consequences

| Situation/Event | Possible Emotion | Consequence |
| CAUSE | REACTION | ACTION TAKEN |

1. _____   _____

2. _____   _____

3. _____   _____

Identifying Situations: Emotions/ Consequences This exercise defines the role of emotions in social interaction. It makes explicit what is generally implicit and obvious to most normally developing children. The sheets need to be customized to the child's actions and behaviors, and the resultant emotions from those behaviors.

This form accompanies *Teach Me Language*. Complete instructions on its use are in Chapter 2 of *Teach Me Language*. Copyright © 1997 SKF Books.

Social Language • 29

Problems, People's Reactions & Solutions

Read about each situation, then answer the questions.

_____

_____

| What is/was the problem? | _____ |

| Who or what caused the problem? | — | Who did the problem affect or bother? | _____ |

| How did it affect _____? | _____ |

| How can the problem be solved? | Solution: _____ |

| How else can the problem be solved? | Another Solution: _____ |

Problems, People's Reactions & Solutions This exercise teaches the relationship between events and people's emotional reactions. The child needs to know why people become angry with him/her and how the child can prevent or decrease the number of unpleasant episodes. This sheet must be customized to the child using situations in which the child 1) makes someone angry; and 2) makes someone sad.

This form accompanies Teach Me Language. Complete instructions on its use are in Chapter 2 of Teach Me Language.
Copyright © 1997 SKF Books.

Identifying If A Situation is Safe or Dangerous

Read each sentence. If the sentence is talking about something dangerous, write "dangerous" on the line. If the sentence is talking about something safe, write "safe" on the line.

Situation   Safe or Dangerous?

_____   _____

_____   _____

_____   _____

_____   _____

_____   _____

Identifying If A Situation is Safe or Dangerous This exercise teaches the child to differentiate safe from dangerous. It is important to use dangers in the child's environment in order to make the drill meaningful. This drill alone will not prevent the child from doing dangerous activities; however, it will start to get the child to think about the categories of safe and dangerous. This drill is a good companion to actual safety training but will not replace intensive lessons on traffic safety, etc. Once the child identifies safe from dangerous, attempt to ask why something is safe or is dangerous. This part of the exercise will require much prompting because the child must have an understanding of Why/Because in order to answer the safety questions.

This form accompanies *Teach Me Language*. Complete instructions on its use are in Chapter 2 of *Teach Me Language*. Copyright © 1997 SKF Books.

Social Language • 31

Identifying If There is a Problem

Read each sentence. If the sentence is talking about a problem, write "problem" on the line. If there is no problem, write "no problem".

Situation	Problem or No Problem?
_____	_____
_____	_____
_____	_____
_____	_____
_____	_____

Identifying If There is a Problem This exercise works on the child's ability to identify problems and solutions. Once the child has completed this exercise with prompting, the therapist should fade out the prompts. Eventually the exercise sheet should be faded and the child should do this exercise orally. As the child becomes more familiar with this drill, the parents should use this same structure to point out problems in the child's natural environment and have the child come up with solutions and do them. *Note: It is important to relate "problem" to danger and "no problem" to being safe (wherever appropriate); however, the child must learn that danger is always a problem, but problems do not always refer to danger. This concept is a difficult one that, over time, the child can be taught.*

This form accompanies Teach Me Language. Complete instructions on its use are in Chapter 2 of Teach Me Language.
Copyright © 1997 SKF Books.

Deciding What To Do

_____

First, STOP AND THINK

What was I asked to do? _____

Next, ASK MYSELF SOME QUESTIONS

Questions   Answers

_____   _____

_____   _____

_____   _____

Then, THINK AND DECIDE WHAT TO DO

What I know: _____

Decide what to do: _____

_____

Deciding What To Do This exercise works on the child's critical thinking skills. The drill teaches the child how to weigh various situations and makes the thinking process explicit. The objective is that this technique will be internalized eventually; however, this may take a long time for most children and some children may always have some trouble with critical thought.

This form accompanies *Teach Me Language*. Complete instructions on its use are in Chapter 2 of *Teach Me Language*. Copyright © 1997 SKF Books.

Problem/Solutions

Problem: _____

_____

Solution: (Prompt) _____

Question probes: _____ (Prompt) _____

_____

(Prompt) _____

Problem: _____

_____

Solution: (Prompt) _____

Question probes: _____ (Prompt) _____

_____

(Prompt) _____

Problem: _____

_____

Solution: (Prompt) _____

Question probes: _____ (Prompt) _____

_____

(Prompt) _____

Problem/Solutions This exercise introduces problems and their solutions. It sets up a formal structure that the child should learn to better understand social rules. To help the child understand this drill, it is very important to customize the examples to situations that arise in the child's life where s/he breaks rules that are often taken for granted as being common sense. The more relevant and realistic the situations, the faster the child will come to understand the concept. This exercise will have to be heavily prompted by the therapist at first; however, once the child understands the drill, the therapist should fade the prompts.

This form accompanies Teach Me Language. Complete instructions on its use are in Chapter 2 of Teach Me Language.
Copyright © 1997 SKF Books.

Identifying "Trouble" and Generating Solutions

Read each problem. Tell what "trouble" each problem causes. Then give a solution to the problem.

Situation   Trouble the Problem Causes

If: _____   Then: _____

    _____   _____

So, Solution: _____

Situation   Trouble the Problem Causes

If: _____   Then: _____

    _____   _____

So, Solution: _____

Identifying "Trouble" and Generating Solutions This exercise structures a critical thinking process that the child should learn in order to understand social rules. It may take a very long time for the child to do this on his/her own. The goal is for the child to eventually generalize this form of critical thinking to his/her natural environment. In order for the child to understand this drill, it is very important to customize examples of situations that arise in the child's life where s/he breaks rules that we take for granted as being common sense. The more relevant and realistic the situations, the faster the child will come to understand this exercise.

This form accompanies *Teach Me Language*. Complete instructions on its use are in Chapter 2 of *Teach Me Language*.
Copyright © 1997 SKF Books.

Identifying If Someone is Being Made Fun Of

Read about each situation. If the situation shows someone being made fun of or being teased in a mean way, write "being made fun of" or "mean teasing" on the line. If it does not show someone being made fun of, write "not being made fun of" or "no teasing" on the line.

Situation   Being Made Fun of or
                                                                    Not Being Made Fun of?

_____   _____

_____   _____

_____   _____

_____   _____

_____

Identifying If Someone is Being Made Fun Of This exercise structures a critical thinking process that the child should learn in order to understand the social interaction of his/her peers. The goal is for the child to be able to recognize when this occurs in his/her natural environment. In order for the child to understand this drill, it is very important to customize situations that arise in the child's life where someone is made fun of. The more relevant and realistic the situations, the faster the child will come to understand this exercise.

This form accompanies Teach Me Language. Complete instructions on its use are in Chapter 2 of Teach Me Language. Copyright © 1997 SKF Books.

Identifying If Something Said is Nice Or Mean

Read each sentence that is "said". Write down if it is a "nice" thing to say or a "mean" thing to say. Then tell if you can "say" it or if you "don't say" it.

What is Said	Nice or Mean?	Say or Don't Say?
_____	_____	_____
_____	_____	_____
_____	_____	_____
_____	_____	_____
_____	_____	_____

Identifying If Something Said is Nice Or Mean This exercise teaches the child to judge whether the person s/he is speaking to is being nice or mean. The exercise should be customized to the child so that experiences from the child's environment are reflected in the exercise. Aside from particular words that are mean or nice, voice inflection also determines whether something said is nice or mean. This drill should be done at first without mean or nice voice inflection. Once the child learns to identify nice from mean in terms of content, then the drill must be done using the same phrases but varying the voice inflection.

This form accompanies *Teach Me Language*. Complete instructions on its use are in Chapter 2 of *Teach Me Language*. Copyright © 1997 SKF Books.

Multiple Opinions

My opinions about: _____

My favorite _____

I like _____

I don't like _____

I believe that _____

I think the best _____

I feel that _____

I think that _____

I don't think that _____

In my opinion _____

I can't stand _____

One of the worst _____

Multiple Opinions This drill has the child formulate and express opinions on one particular topic. Food is a good topic to begin with since most children have opinions about food. This sheet uses several different ways to convey the same negative or positive opinions. It is important for the child to know these different words so that they can understand them when other children and adults use them.

This form accompanies Teach Me Language. Complete instructions on its use are in Chapter 2 of Teach Me Language.
Copyright © 1997 SKF Books.

Opinions and Supporting Reasons: Food

Choose 3 _____:

Food	Opinion		Supporting Reason		
_____ _____ _____	like	don't like	good delicious juicy sweet	sour awful bad too spicy	crunchy gooey cold hot
_____ _____ _____	like	don't like	good delicious juicy sweet	sour awful bad too spicy	crunchy gooey cold hot
_____ _____ _____	like	don't like	good delicious juicy sweet	sour awful bad too spicy	crunchy gooey cold hot

_____

_____

Opinions and Supporting Reasons: Food The following exercise gives the child a structure within which to voice an opinion and sets up a set of reasons from which to choose. It is important to make sure the topics chosen are familiar to the child and that the child has an opinion about them. Food is a particularly good topic since children have definite preferences in this area.

This form accompanies *Teach Me Language*. Complete instructions on its use are in Chapter 2 of *Teach Me Language*. Copyright © 1997 SKF Books.

Opinions and Supporting Reasons: Movies

Choose 3 _____:

Movies	Opinion	Supporting Reason

_____   like   don't like   boring   exciting
_____   scary   funny
_____   bad   good
                                               too hard to   entertaining
                                               understand   (fun to watch)

_____   like   don't like   boring   exciting
_____   scary   funny
_____   bad   good
                                               too hard to   entertaining
                                               understand   (fun to watch)

_____   like   don't like   boring   exciting
_____   scary   funny
_____   bad   good
                                               too hard to   entertaining
                                               understand   (fun to watch)

_____

_____

Opinions and Supporting Reasons: Movies This exercise gives the child a structure within which to voice an opinion and provides a set of reasons from which to choose. It is important to make sure the topics chosen are familiar to the child and that the child has an opinion about them. The topic, "Movies" is more difficult than food, but is a good topic since most typically developing children have opinions about movies.

This form accompanies Teach Me Language. Complete instructions on its use are in Chapter 2 of Teach Me Language.
Copyright © 1997 SKF Books.

Fact Or Opinion?

Read each statement about the topic or event. Tell whether it is a fact or an opinion. Then state one more fact about the topic/event and give your own opinion about the topic/event.

Topic or Event: _____   Fact or Opinion?

_____   _____

_____   _____

_____   _____

_____   _____

Fact about: _____   _____

_____

My Opinion about: _____   _____

_____

Fact Or Opinion? This exercise teaches a child the difference between a person's opinion and a factual statement. The topic should interest the child and be a topic the child knows something about. The first part of the exercise has the child differentiate between opinion and fact, the second part gives the child the opportunity to tell the therapist a fact about the topic and give his/her opinion about it. The category of movies the child enjoys is an example of a good topic to choose, even if s/he does not fully understand the movie.

This form accompanies *Teach Me Language*. Complete instructions on its use are in Chapter 2 of *Teach Me Language*.
Copyright © 1997 SKF Books.

My Opinions (About School)

My Opinions About School

In school the thing I like to do best is _____

My favorite thing to do at recess is _____

At school I don't like to _____

When they have _____ for lunch I don't like to eat it.

I think that school is _____

Facts about my school:

The name of my school is _____ Elementary.

Lots of kids go to my school.

There is hot lunch at my school.

The playground at school is large.

There are many classrooms at my school.

My Opinions (About School) This exercise is designed to show the child the difference between opinions and facts by having the child list his/her opinions above a list of facts about his/her school. Once the child lists his/her opinions, then the child should read through the facts about the school. The therapist should then read an opinion or a fact and ask the child to identify what the statement is i.e. fact or opinion.

This form accompanies Teach Me Language. Complete instructions on its use are in Chapter 2 of Teach Me Language.
Copyright © 1997 SKF Books.

My Opinions (About Movies)

My Opinions About Movies

My favorite movie is _____. I like it because _____.

The scariest movie I have ever seen is _____.

The funniest movie I have ever seen is _____.

I don't like _____ because _____.

_____ is a good movie.

Facts about movies:

Movies are about people, places, and things.

You can see movies at the movie theater.

> The Lion King is about Simba and Nala.
> Pocahontas is about Pocahontas and John Smith.
> Snow White is about Snow White and the Seven Dwarfs.
> Beauty and the Beast is about Belle and the Beast.

My Opinions (Movies) This exercise is designed to show the child the difference between opinions and facts by having the child list his/her opinions above a list of facts about movies. Once the child lists his/her opinions, then the child should read through the facts about movies. The therapist should then read an opinion or a fact and ask the child to identify what the statement is i.e. fact or opinion.

This form accompanies *Teach Me Language*. Complete instructions on its use are in Chapter 2 of *Teach Me Language*.
Copyright © 1997 SKF Books.

3 General Knowledge
Forms

- Outline for Topical Information
- Simple Child - Generated Outline
- Simple Outline with Elaborative Statement
- Multi-Paragraph Outline
- Oral Definitions: Animals
- Animal Grid Fill-In (Introduction to Animal Comparisons)
- True or False? (1)
- True or False? (2)
- Outline For Topical Information
- Simple Child - Generated Outline
- Simple Outline with Elaborative Statement
- Multi-Paragraph Outline
- Oral Definitions: Occupations
- Occupation Grid Fill-In
- Who Would Say This?
- What Would They Say?
- Current Topics
- Making Comparisons
- Grid Comparison
- +/- Comparison
- Sport Comparisons Using "Both"
- General Comparisons (1)
- General Comparisons (2)

Forms in this chapter accompany Teach Me Language. Complete instructions on their use are in Chapter 3 of Teach Me Language. Copyright © 1997 SKF Books.

Outline For Topical Information

Topic: _____

Main Idea: _____

Details: _____

_____

_____

_____

_____

_____

_____

Outline For Topical Information This exercise teaches the child 1) how to learn from the written word, and 2) how to distinguish between main idea and detail. To make this drill easy or intermediate, the outline should be completed by the therapist before the session. To make this drill more difficult, the child should fill in the details with the therapist during the drill. First, the child reads the paragraph with the therapist. Then the therapist uses the outline to help the child comprehend and talk about the paragraph.

This form accompanies *Teach Me Language*. Complete instructions on its use are in Chapter 3 of *Teach Me Language*.
Copyright © 1997 SKF Books.

Simple Child - Generated Outline

Topic: _____

Main Idea: _____

Tell me about _____

Details: _____

              _____

              _____

Simple Child - Generated Outline This exercise teaches the child how to comprehend the written word and differentiate main idea and detail. This outline should be completed by the child during the session after the therapist has gone over the easy and intermediate therapist-generated outline with the child. First the child reads the paragraph. Then the child dictates the information to the therapist. At first, the child should be expected to give one word only. Eventually, the child should be able to tell the therapist about the topic in full sentences by using these single words as prompts. Once the child has mastered this skill, s/he should be given the opportunity to write a short paragraph based on his/her outline.

This form accompanies *Teach Me Language*. Complete instructions on its use are in Chapter 3 of *Teach Me Language*.
Copyright © 1997 SKF Books.

Simple Outline with Elaborative Statement

Topic: _____

Tell me about: _____

Main Idea: _____

Detail: _____

Detail: _____

Detail: _____

Detail: _____

Simple Outline with Elaborative Statement This outline, like the simple outline, should be completed by the child during the session. First the child should read the paragraph with the therapist. Then the child should dictate the words to be written on the outline to the therapist. The child should give a detail and then elaborate on that detail. Once the child has mastered the Outline with Elaborative Statement, s/he should be given the opportunity to write a short paragraph based on his/her outline.

This form accompanies *Teach Me Language*. Complete instructions on its use are in Chapter 3 of *Teach Me Language*.
Copyright © 1997 SKF Books.

Multi-Paragraph Outline

Topic: _____

General Info: _____
_____
_____

1. Topic: _____

   Details: _____
   _____
   _____

2. Topic: _____

   Details: _____
   _____
   _____

3. Topic: _____

   Details: _____
   _____
   _____

4. Topic: _____

   Details: _____
   _____
   _____

Multi-Paragraph Outline This advanced exercise should be introduced only when the child has a firm grasp of the "Simple Outline with Elaborate Statement". After the child reads the paragraph with the therapist, s/he should dictate the relevant information to the therapist. The therapist should ask questions when the child is stuck. The child should give the therapist 1) the topic, and a few details about the topic, and 2) examples of the topic. Those examples become the main idea for the smaller paragraphs. Then, the child should be asked to come up with three details for each secondary topic. Using this completed outline, the child should be able to talk about the topic.

This form accompanies *Teach Me Language*. Complete instructions on its use are in Chapter 3 of *Teach Me Language*. Copyright © 1997 SKF Books.

Oral Definitions: Animals

Give a definition of each animal by filling in the blanks.

Animals: _____, _____, _____, _____

1. A _____ is a _____ with _____.

2. A _____ is a _____ that has _____.

3. A _____ is a _____ with _____.

4. A _____ is a _____ that has _____.

Oral Definitions: Animals The oral definition sheet should be introduced to the child once s/he has learned four animals. With every additional animal, the oral definition exercise can be used to learn about the new animal and maintain the information the child has acquired earlier about other animals. By combining animals that the child knows well with animals that s/he does not, the information is easily maintained. A few of the definitions are very easy and, therefore, highly motivating.

This form accompanies *Teach Me Language*. Complete instructions on its use are in Chapter 3 of *Teach Me Language*.
Copyright © 1997 SKF Books.

Animal Grid Fill-In (Introduction to Animal Comparisons)

Fill in the blank boxes with what you know about each animal.

Animal			
is			
has			
lives			
eats			

Animal Grid Fill-In The Animal Grid Fill-In sheet should be introduced to the child once s/he has learned three animals. This exercise is somewhat harder than the definitions because the child must give four details about each animal; however, once the child understands the below structure, each animal will become progressively easier. This exercise can maintain the information the child has acquired previously by mixing newly introduced animals with familiar animals. Using this strategy should make the drill motivating because a few of the animals will be very easy to describe. Once the child becomes good at completing the grid, this exercise can be substituted with a more challenging comparison drill (see the section on comparisons in this chapter).

This form accompanies *Teach Me Language*. Complete instructions on its use are in Chapter 3 of *Teach Me Language*.
Copyright © 1997 SKF Books.

True or False? (1)

Statement   If false, why...?

1. _____   _____

2. _____   _____

3. _____   _____

4. _____   _____

5. _____   _____

6. _____   _____

True or False? (1) The True or False exercise can include any information the child has **already learned**. The goal of this exercise is to hone the child's ability to differentiate between true and false because this ability to differentiate is a cornerstone to critical thinking. The True or False exercise is NOT designed to teach the child new information; rather, it is meant to be used with information that the child already has learned.

This form accompanies *Teach Me Language*. Complete instructions on its use are in Chapter 3 of *Teach Me Language*.
Copyright © 1997 SKF Books.

True or False? (2)

Statement   If false, why...?

1. _____   _____

2. _____   _____

3. _____   _____

4. _____   _____

5. _____   _____

6. _____   _____

True or False? (2) This True or False exercise is a variation of the general true or false exercises. This exercise must include information the child knows well because the goal here is to strengthen the child's ability to discern between words that represent relative amounts such as most, much, or all. The goal of this exercise is to improve the child's ability to differentiate between these subtle true and false statements. This variation should only be done with the child once s/he understands the first True or False exercise very well.

This form accompanies Teach Me Language. *Complete instructions on its use are in Chapter 3 of* Teach Me Language.
Copyright © 1997 SKF Books.

Outline For Topical Information

Topic: _____

Main Idea: _____

Details: _____

_____

_____

_____

_____

_____

_____

Outline For Topical Information This exercise teaches the child how to comprehend text and differentiate between main idea and detail. The outline should be completed by the therapist before the session begins. First, the child reads the paragraph. Then, the therapist uses the outline to help the child comprehend and talk about the paragraph. Eventually the child should be able to tell the therapist what information should be included in the outline.

This form accompanies *Teach Me Language*. Complete instructions on its use are in Chapter 3 of *Teach Me Language*.
Copyright © 1997 SKF Books.

Simple Child - Generated Outline

Topic: _____

Main Idea: _____

Tell me about _____

Details: _____

_____

_____

Simple Child - Generated Outline This exercise teaches the child how to organize information. The outline should be completed by the child during the session. First, the child reads the paragraph. Then, s/he dictates the information to the therapist. Initially, the child should only be expected to give one word. Eventually, the child should be able to tell the therapist about the topic in complete sentences by using these words as prompts. Once the child has mastered this exercise, s/he should be given the opportunity to write a short paragraph based on his/her outline.

This form accompanies *Teach Me Language*. Complete instructions on its use are in Chapter 3 of *Teach Me Language*.
Copyright © 1997 SKF Books.

Simple Outline with Elaborative Statement

Topic: _____

Tell me about _____

Main Idea: _____

    Detail: _____

    Detail: _____

    Detail: _____

    Detail: _____

Simple Outline with Elaborative Statement This exercise teaches the child how to comprehend and organize information. This outline, like the simple outline, should be completed by the child during the session. First, the child reads the paragraph. Then, the child should dictate the information to the therapist. The child should give a detail from the paragraph and then elaborate on that detail. Once the child has mastered the outline with elaborative statement, s/he should be given the opportunity to write a short paragraph based on his/her outline.

This form accompanies *Teach Me Language*. Complete instructions on its use are in Chapter 3 of *Teach Me Language*. Copyright © 1997 SKF Books.

Multi-Paragraph Outline

Topic: _____

General Info: _____
_____
_____

1. Topic: _____

   Details: _____
   _____
   _____

2. Topic: _____

   Details: _____
   _____
   _____

3. Topic: _____

   Details: _____
   _____
   _____

4. Topic: _____

   Details: _____
   _____
   _____

Multi-Paragraph Outline This exercise teaches the child how to comprehend and organize information from a written text. The outline should be completed by the child during the session. First, the child reads the paragraph. Then, the child dictates the information to the therapist. The child should tell the therapist the topic of the paragraph, and give a few details about the topic. Then, the child should be prompted to give examples of the topic. Those examples become the main idea for the smaller paragraphs. Next, the child should be asked to come up with three details for each secondary topic. Finally, the child should be able to talk about the topic using this outline.

This form accompanies *Teach Me Language*. Complete instructions on its use are in Chapter 3 of *Teach Me Language*. Copyright © 1997 SKF Books.

Oral Definitions: Occupations

Give a definition of each occupation by filling in the blanks.

Occupation: _____, _____, _____, _____.

1. A _____ is a _____ who _____.

2. A _____ is a _____ who _____.

3. A _____ is a _____ who _____.

4. A _____ is a _____ who _____.

Oral Definitions: Occupations The oral definition sheet can be introduced to the child once s/he has studied four occupations. With every additional occupation introduced, the oral definition exercise can be used to solidify the new occupation and maintain the information the child has already acquired. By adding occupations that the child knows well, with occupations that s/he does not, the information is easily remembered and the more familiar definitions become very easy and highly motivating.

This form accompanies *Teach Me Language*. Complete instructions on its use are in Chapter 3 of *Teach Me Language*.
Copyright © 1997 SKF Books.

Occupation Grid Fill-In (Introduction to Occupation Comparisons)

Fill in the blank boxes with what you know about each occupation.

Job			
is a person who			
works			
uses			
wears/does			

Occupation Grid Fill-In The Occupation Grid Fill-In sheet should be introduced to the child once s/he has learned three occupations. The child has already been introduced to the structure when learning about animals. The addition of occupations the child knows well (to ones that s/he is just learning), easily maintains the familiar information and highly motivates the child since the child finds part of the exercise easy. Once the child is good at this easy comparison, more difficult comparisons can be substituted (see the end of this chapter).

This form accompanies *Teach Me Language*. Complete instructions on its use are in Chapter 3 of *Teach Me Language*. Copyright © 1997 SKF Books.

Who Would Say This?

Read the directions:

You have learned about a _____, _____, _____, _____, _____, _____, _____, _____.

You should know what each person might say.

Read what is said and write down WHO would say it on the line.

Who?	Says What?
1._____	"Don't eat candy."
2._____	"Don't play with matches."
3._____	"Do your homework."
4._____	"May I take your order?"
5._____	"Brush your teeth".
6._____	"Let me take your temperature."
7._____	"Where does it hurt?"
8._____	"Pass me the hammer."

Who Would Say This? This exercise has the child identify the occupation based on what a member of that occupation would say. This drill should be introduced only when the child has learned about eight occupations from the paragraphs. Some occupations are harder to identify than others. The easy questions must be included to give the child the opportunity to successfully answer some of the questions unprompted. If the child has difficulty giving an answer, it is important to prompt the child to guarantee success.

This form accompanies *Teach Me Language*. Complete instructions on its use are in Chapter 3 of *Teach Me Language*.
Copyright © 1997 SKF Books.

General Knowledge • 59

What Would They Say?

Read the directions:

You have learned about a _____, _____, _____, _____, _____, _____, _____, _____.

You should know who says what.

Read the name of the job and write down what each occupation would say on the line.

Who?   Says What?

1. Doctor   _____

2. Dentist   _____

3. Fire fighter   _____

4. Waiter   _____

5. Clerk   _____

6. Carpenter   _____

7. Chef   _____

8. Policeman   _____

What Would They Say? This exercise is designed to take the knowledge the child has gained from the occupation paragraphs and make him/her critically think about what members of each occupation say. This is a difficult exercise because the child has to think about what members of the occupation do, and then think of something that those members would say that is relevant to the occupation.

This form accompanies *Teach Me Language*. Complete instructions on its use are in Chapter 3 of *Teach Me Language*.
Copyright © 1997 SKF Books.

Current Topics

Date   Theme   Topic   Information Child Should Know
(for all topics)

Current Topics This record sheet is designed to give the therapist a sense of how quickly or slowly the child is progressing through the paragraphs, and which paragraphs have been covered and need to be reviewed.

This form accompanies *Teach Me Language*. Complete instructions on its use are in Chapter 3 of *Teach Me Language*.
Copyright © 1997 SKF Books.

Making Comparisons

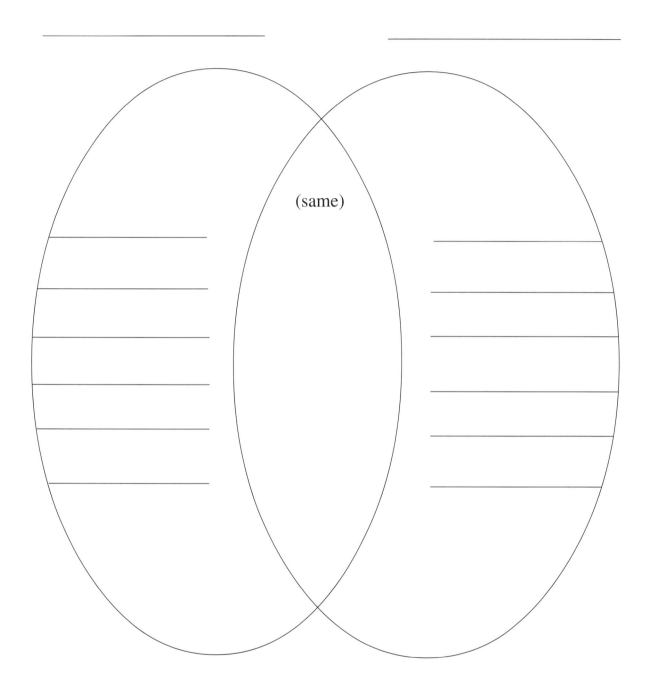

Making Comparisons The Venn Diagram Comparison exercise gives a visual representation of the concept of same and different. The first time the child does this exercise, the therapist should have all the descriptors of each animal listed. The therapist should direct the child to circle the descriptors that are the same for each animal. Then the therapist can draw an arrow into the middle (while the child observes) and write the common descriptor that the child has just circled in the intersecting circle.

This form accompanies *Teach Me Language*. Complete instructions on its use are in Chapter 3 of *Teach Me Language*. Copyright © 1997 SKF Books.

Grid Comparison (Animal, Occupation Sport, etc...)

_____ Comparison

Fill in the grid for each _____
Then circle the features that are the same for each _____

Feature Compared		

Grid Comparison This exercise is an elaboration of the easier comparison. It is introduced to the child in much the same way as the easier grid. This Grid Fill-In sheet should be introduced to the child once s/he has learned two animals, occupations or sports from the medium or difficult paragraphs.

This form accompanies *Teach Me Language*. Complete instructions on its use are in Chapter 3 of *Teach Me Language*.
Copyright © 1997 SKF Books.

General Knowledge • 63

+/- Comparison (Animal, Occupation, Sport, etc...)

Look at each _____ fact.
Put a "+" in the box under the correct _____ for each true fact.
Put a "-" in the box under the correct _____ for each fact that is false.
Then circle the "+" or true features that are the same for each _____ .

Fact		

+/- Comparison This exercise is introduced to the child in the same way as the +/- Occupation Comparison. This Grid Fill-In sheet should be used once the child has learned two different types of sport, animal or occupation.

This form accompanies *Teach Me Language*. Complete instructions on its use are in Chapter 3 of *Teach Me Language*.
Copyright © 1997 SKF Books.

Sport Comparisons Using "Both"

Tell which sport _____ (or Both) goes with each of the following:

What   Which Sport

_____   _____

_____   _____

_____   _____

_____   _____

_____   _____

_____   _____

Sport Comparisons Using "Both" This exercise should accompany the topic of sports and should be given to the child after s/he has learned about two sports (from the sport paragraphs). The exercise helps reinforce what has been learned and maintains the role of the word "both", thereby widening the type of comparison the child can make. The Sport Comparison exercise illustrates the way to customize an exercise for a specific area of interest. The same structure can be used for different types of interests e.g. dance, gymnastics, musical instruments, art.

This form accompanies *Teach Me Language*. Complete instructions on its use are in Chapter 3 of *Teach Me Language*.
Copyright © 1997 SKF Books.

General Comparisons (1)

How are a _____ and _____ the same?

They both...
_____

How are a _____ and _____ different?

A _____

But

A _____

How are a _____ and _____ the same?

They both...
_____

How are a _____ and _____ different?

A _____

But

A _____

General Comparisons (1) This comparison exercise is more difficult than the previous comparison exercises because the child must find similarities and differences without being directed by the structure of the exercise. There are many correct answers to this exercise which gives the child the opportunity to be successful. Once the child understands this exercise well, then it is important to point out the most obvious answers to the child (even if the child correctly gives another answer).

This form accompanies *Teach Me Language*. Complete instructions on its use are in Chapter 3 of *Teach Me Language*.
Copyright © 1997 SKF Books.

General Knowledge • 66

General Comparisons (2)

Look at this comparison form.
Answer the questions below.

How _____ the same?

    They Both...

_____

_____

_____

_____

How _____ different?

_____

_____

_____

_____

_____

General Comparisons (2) Prerequisite: The child should be able to complete a grid comparison before this General Comparison sheet is introduced. This comparison exercise is much harder than the first general comparison exercise because the child must find as many similarities and differences as s/he can. This exercise is worth doing over a period of years because it works on the child's logical and critical thinking skills. Once the child is comfortable with general comparisons, this sheet should be removed. At this point, the child should be able to compare two subjects without using any visual prompts.

This form accompanies *Teach Me Language*. Complete instructions on its use are in Chapter 3 of *Teach Me Language*.
Copyright © 1997 SKF Books.

4 Grammar and Syntax
Forms

- Classifying Pronouns
- Pronoun Referents Exercise
- Super Sentences
- Identifying Phrases

Forms in this chapter accompany Teach Me Language. Complete instructions on their use are in Chapter 4 of Teach Me Language.
Copyright © 1997 SKF Books.

Classifying Pronouns

Write each word or phrase in the correct pronoun box.

Words: _____

he	she	it	we	they

Classifying Pronouns This exercise teaches the child to classify pronouns. This skill is important for reading comprehension. The child should write each word under the appropriate pronoun.

This form accompanies *Teach Me Language*. Complete instructions on its use are in Chapter 4 of *Teach Me Language*. Copyright © 1997 SKF Books.

Pronoun Referents Exercise

A PRONOUN takes the place of a noun.
Circle the noun or nouns that the underlined pronoun refers to. Draw an arrow from the pronoun to its referent.

1. _____
   _____

2. _____
   _____

3. _____
   _____

4. _____
   _____

5. _____
   _____

Pronoun Referents This exercise teaches the child about the relationship between pronouns and nouns. If the child does not understand the role of pronouns, it will be very difficult for him/her to comprehend text and will hamper comprehension of simple conversation.

This form accompanies *Teach Me Language*. Complete instructions on its use are in Chapter 4 of *Teach Me Language*.
Copyright © 1997 SKF Books.

Super Sentences

Building a Sentence:

Fill in the boxes with words to make a long sentence.

	describing words	who or what?	does what?	where?	when?

	describing words	who or what?	does what?	where?	when?

	describing words	who or what?	does what?	where?	when?

Super Sentences This exercise teaches children the parts of a sentence and gives them the opportunity to create their own sentence in a structured way. The goal of this exercise is for the child to start to understand the function of each part of the sentence so s/he will be able to understand and create longer sentences.

This form accompanies *Teach Me Language*. Complete instructions on its use are in Chapter 4 of *Teach Me Language*. Copyright © 1997 SKF Books.

Grammar & Syntax • 71

Identifying Phrases

Read each phrase. Put an X under what each phrase tells about.

	Who/What?	Did What?	Where?	When?
1. _____				
2. _____				
3. _____				
4. _____				
5. _____				
6. _____				
7. _____				
8. _____				
9. _____				
10. _____				

Write a phrase that tells *who or what* _____.

Write a phrase that tells *did what* _____.

Write a phrase that tells *where* _____.

Write a phrase that tells *when* _____.

Identifying Phrases This exercise teaches children to identify the various parts of a sentence by their function. This is another way to work on WH questions visually in order to improve the child's auditory understanding.

This form accompanies *Teach Me Language*. Complete instructions on its use are in Chapter 4 of *Teach Me Language*. Copyright © 1997 SKF Books.

5 Advanced Language Development

Forms

- Easy Story Writing
- Intermediate Story Writing
- Difficult Story Writing
- Advanced Story Writing
- Easy Story Pre-Writing
- Difficult Story Pre-Writing
- Advanced Story Pre-Writing
- Writing a Topic Sentence
- Outline for Paragraph Writing & Topical Conversation - Easy
- Outline for Paragraph Writing and Topical Conversation - Intermediate
- Outline for Paragraph Writing and Topical Conversation - Advanced
- Writing a Paragraph
- Developing Your Story (Introductory Paragraph)
- Developing Your Story - Paragraph 2
- Developing Your Story - Paragraph 3
- Developing Your Story - Paragraph 4
- Finding the Main Idea
- Sentence Starters For Descriptive Topic Sentences & Detail Sentences of Support
- Two-Column Notes
- Letter Template
- What I Did Today: (What Did You Do Today?)
- Daily Routine Sheet (Recall of Day)

Forms in this chapter accompany Teach Me Language. Complete instructions on their use are in Chapter 5 of Teach Me Language. Copyright © 1997 SKF Books.

Advanced Language Development • 74

Easy Story Writing

Subject/Title: _____

Once upon a time there was a _____

_____name was _____

One day _____

First, _____

Next, _____

Last, _____

Easy Story Writing This is the easiest story template. It should be completed by the therapist with the child helping until the child understands the structure. The child should work on the easy story template until s/he can complete it, with no prompts whatsoever. Eventually, the child should be able to tell a story orally without using the sheet.

This form accompanies *Teach Me Language*. Complete instructions on its use are in Chapter 5 of *Teach Me Language*.
Copyright © 1997 SKF Books.

Intermediate Story Writing

Subject/Title: _____

Once upon a time there was a _____

_____ name was _____

One day _____

_____

First, _____

_____

Next, _____

_____

Last, _____

_____

Intermediate Story Writing The intermediate story template should be introduced once the child understands the structure of the easy template. The intermediate template introduces the idea of elaborative descriptive sentences (using another sentence to elaborate on the original sentence in a descriptive way). The child should work on this template until it is easy to complete independently.

This form accompanies *Teach Me Language*. Complete instructions on its use are in Chapter 5 of *Teach Me Language*.
Copyright © 1997 SKF Books.

Difficult Story Writing

(Subject/Title) _____

_____

_____

_____

First, _____ and _____

_____

_____

After _____

_____ and _____

_____

Last _____ and _____

_____

_____

Difficult story template This template should be introduced once the child understands the structure of the intermediate template. The difficult template introduces the idea of conversation within a story and emphasizes its structure.

This form accompanies *Teach Me Language*. Complete instructions on its use are in Chapter 5 of *Teach Me Language*. Copyright © 1997 SKF Books.

Advanced Story Writing

(Subject/Title) _____

_____
_____
_____
_____
_____

First, _____ and _____
_____
_____

After _____
_____ and _____
_____

Last _____ and _____
_____
_____

Advanced story template The advanced story template should be introduced once the child understands the structure of the difficult template. This template introduces the idea of character development within a story and builds upon the structure of the difficult story template. As the child becomes better at story writing, it is important to introduce other ways to start a story besides "Once upon a time" (e.g. One day...).

This form accompanies *Teach Me Language*. Complete instructions on its use are in Chapter 5 of *Teach Me Language*.
Copyright © 1997 SKF Books.

Easy Story Pre-Writing

Subject/Title: _____

Characters: _____

_____

_____

Setting: _____

_____

_____

_____

Time: _____

_____

_____

_____

Easy Pre-writing Template The easy pre-writing template should be introduced once the child understands the structure of the easiest story template. Story Pre-Writing teaches the child to make an outline of the story that s/he will write. In this easy form, the outline has the child come up with the names of the characters, the setting and when the story takes place. This pre-writing sheet is for a story titled "Two Girls at the Park".

This form accompanies *Teach Me Language*. Complete instructions on its use are in Chapter 5 of *Teach Me Language*.
Copyright © 1997 SKF Books.

Difficult Story Pre-Writing

Story Title: _____

Characters: _____ | _____

(how old)

(what they like)

(a descriptive e.g.
big, tall, small)

Setting: _____

_____

_____

_____

Time: _____

_____

_____

_____

Difficult Pre-writing template. The difficult pre-writing template should be introduced once the child understands the structure of the easiest pre-writing template. In this form, the outline has the child describe his/her characters, elaborate on the setting and give a more in-depth idea of when the story takes place. *Note: Either the therapist gives the topic, or the child chooses a topic. If the child chooses, it is important that the child suggests a different topic each time the exercise is done.*

This form accompanies *Teach Me Language*. Complete instructions on its use are in Chapter 5 of *Teach Me Language*.
Copyright © 1997 SKF Books.

Advanced Story Pre-writing

Story Title: _____

Characters: _____
　　　　　　　_____ | _____
　　　　　　　_____ |

Setting: _____
_____
_____

Time: _____
_____

STORY and SEQUENCE:

Paragraph 1: from above

Paragraph 2: First _____ and _____

Paragraph 3: After _____, _____ and _____

Paragraph 4: Last _____ and _____

Advanced Pre-writing template. The Advanced Pre-writing template should be introduced once the child understands the structure of the preceding pre-writing templates. This work sheet actually constitutes an entire outline of a story from a description of the characters, an elaboration on the setting, an idea of when the story takes place to the actual sequence of events. At this stage, the child should be filling out his/her own pre-writing form.

This form accompanies *Teach Me Language*. Complete instructions on its use are in Chapter 5 of *Teach Me Language*.
Copyright © 1997 SKF Books.

Writing a Topic Sentence

For each topic below, write 2 different topic sentences.

Topic: _____

Topic Sentence #1: _____

Topic Sentence #2: _____

Topic: _____

Topic Sentence #1: _____

Topic Sentence #2: _____

Topic: _____

Topic Sentence #1: _____

Topic Sentence #2: _____

Writing a Topic Sentence Exercise This exercise teaches the child to write a topic sentence. After the child has read the script about topic sentences (on the preceding page), the therapist gives a topic and the child writes two topic sentences. At first, the therapist will need to prompt the child to complete the exercise; however, once the child understands how to complete this exercise, s/he should complete it independently. Eventually, the therapist should remove the sheet altogether and ask the child to orally create a topic sentence.

This form accompanies *Teach Me Language*. Complete instructions on its use are in Chapter 5 of *Teach Me Language*.
Copyright © 1997 SKF Books.

Outline for Paragraph Writing & Topical Conversation - Easy

TOPIC: _____
*(what you want
to talk about)*

MAIN IDEA: _____
*(what you want to say
about the topic)*

① _____

DETAILS:
*(the important things
you want to say about
the main idea)*

② _____

③ _____

④ _____

Outline for Paragraph Writing & Topical Conversation - Easy This exercise teaches the child the structure of a paragraph (that a paragraph is about a topic and is made up of a main idea and details). This exercise gives the child a rigid structure with which to organize thoughts. Within this structure, the child will find it easier to be creative.

Outline for Paragraph Writing and Topical Conversation - Intermediate

TOPIC: _____
*(what you want
to talk about)*

MAIN IDEA: _____
*(what you want to say
about the topic)*

① _____

DETAILS: ② _____
*(the important things
you want to say about
the main idea)*

③ _____

④ _____

Outline for Paragraph Writing & Topical Conversation - Intermediate The intermediate level of this exercise teaches the child that within the structure of a paragraph there is room for elaboration. Although the rigid structure is still adhered to, each detail has an elaborative statement (which is typical in paragraphs).

Outline for Paragraph Writing and Topical Conversation - Advanced

TOPIC: _____

MAIN IDEA(S): _____

_____

_____

Paragraph Topic: ① _____

Details: _____

_____

Paragraph Topic: ② _____

Details: _____

_____

Paragraph Topic: ③ _____

Details: _____

_____

Paragraph Topic: ④ _____

Details: _____

_____

Outline for Paragraph Writing & Topical Conversation - Advanced The advanced version of this exercise shows that an essay, report, or paper has a main paragraph which introduces the subject of the paragraphs in the body of the writing, and that each paragraph in the body has its own main idea and details. Elaborative statements can be introduced here as the next step.

This form accompanies *Teach Me Language*. Complete instructions on its use are in Chapter 5 of *Teach Me Language*.
Copyright © 1997 SKF Books.

Writing a Paragraph

TOPIC: _____

Topic Sentence:

(main idea)

_____

3 Supporting Sentences:

(Details)

1. _____

2. _____

3. _____

Concluding Sentence:

(Summary sentence that retells the main idea)

_____

Writing a Paragraph This sheet is designed to make explicit the structure of a paragraph. It will make it easier for the child to write paragraphs and will hopefully improve the child's story writing as well.

This form accompanies *Teach Me Language*. Complete instructions on its use are in Chapter 5 of *Teach Me Language*.
Copyright © 1997 SKF Books.

Developing Your Story (Introductory Paragraph)

Story Title: _____

Introductory Paragraph

Topic Sentence: _____

_____

Supporting Details:
(Character Description - 1st Character)

_____

_____

(Character Description - 2nd Character)

_____

_____

Setting/Time Paragraph

Topic Sentence: _____

_____

Supporting Details:

_____

_____

_____

Developing Your Story (Introductory Paragraph) The following four sheets give the child the opportunity to put all the various parts of a story together in one outline. This sheet lays out the topic sentence in the first paragraph and joins it with character development and elaborative sentences. The following sheets help the child develop the paragraphs within the story.

This form accompanies *Teach Me Language*. Complete instructions on its use are in Chapter 5 of *Teach Me Language*.
Copyright © 1997 SKF Books.

Developing Your Story - Paragraph 2

EVENT PARAGRAPH (1)

Topic Sentence: _____

_____

Supporting Details (3 Sentences of Support):

1. _____

_____

_____

2. _____

_____

_____

3. _____

_____

_____

Developing Your Story - Paragraph 2 This sheet lays out the topic sentence in the second paragraph and joins it with detail sentences which support the topic sentence.

This form accompanies *Teach Me Language*. Complete instructions on its use are in Chapter 5 of *Teach Me Language*. Copyright © 1997 SKF Books.

Developing Your Story - Paragraph 3

EVENT PARAGRAPH (2)

Topic Sentence: _____

Supporting Details (3 Sentences of Support):

1. _____

   _____

   _____

2. _____

   _____

   _____

3. _____

   _____

   _____

Developing Your Story - Paragraph 4 This sheet lays out the topic sentence in the third paragraph and joins it with detail sentences which support the topic sentence.

This form accompanies *Teach Me Language*. Complete instructions on its use are in Chapter 5 of *Teach Me Language*. Copyright © 1997 SKF Books.

Developing Your Story - Paragraph 4

EVENT PARAGRAPH (3)

Topic Sentence: _____

_____

Supporting Details (3 Sentences of Support):

1. _____

_____

_____

_____

2. _____

_____

_____

3. _____

_____

Developing Your Story - Paragraph 4 This sheet lays out the topic sentence in the fourth and concluding paragraph and joins it with detail sentences which support the topic sentence.

Finding the Main Idea

Look at each list. Determine the main idea and the details. Then write a topic sentence for your main idea.

List: _____   Main Idea: _____

_____   *Details:* _____

_____   _____

_____   _____

Topic Sentence: _____

_____

List: _____   Main Idea: _____

_____   *Details:* _____

_____   _____

_____   _____

Topic Sentence: _____

_____

Finding the Main Idea This exercise is designed to work on the comprehension skills of the child without requiring the child to read a paragraph. This sheet can be introduced to the child before the outline for paragraph writing is introduced or once the child knows how to write a simple paragraph.

This form accompanies Teach Me Language. Complete instructions on its use are in Chapter 5 of Teach Me Language.
Copyright © 1997 SKF Books.

Sentence Starters For Descriptive Topic Sentences and Detail Sentences of Support

Topic Sentence: There are many kinds of _____.

Detail Sentences:

    A _____ is a kind of _____.

    One kind of _____ is _____.

    Another kind of _____ is _____.

    _____ is also a kind of _____.

Topic Sentence: A _____ is a _____.
                (that has/with/that can)

Detail Sentences:

    For example, _____ is _____.

    An example of _____ is _____.

    A _____ is an example of _____.

    Another example of _____ is _____.

    _____ is also an example of _____.

Topic Sentence: A _____ is a _____.
                (that has/with/that can)

Detail Sentences:

    One type of _____ is _____.

    A _____ is a type of _____.

    Another type of _____ is _____.

    _____ is also a type of _____.

Sentence Starters For Descriptive Topic Sentences and Detail Sentences of Support This exercise introduces the child to the structure of detail sentences and their relationship to topic sentences. The topic should be one which the child has learned about and knows well. This topic in the example corresponds to a paragraph in the general information chapter.

This form accompanies *Teach Me Language*. Complete instructions on its use are in Chapter 5 of *Teach Me Language*.
Copyright © 1997 SKF Books.

Two-Column Notes

What Is The Text About?

1st Paragraph Topic:	Details:
Main Idea:	

2nd Paragraph Topic:	Details:
Main Idea:	

3rd Paragraph Topic:	Details:
Main Idea:	

Two Column Notes This sheet is designed to help the child comprehend a descriptive paragraph by taking notes from that paragraph in a structured way. The sheet has room for three paragraphs that may be related to one another; however, when the child is learning this skill, each paragraph should be able to stand alone.
There are two columns so the child can glance at the left column and know what the paragraph is about without the details in the right column distracting him/her.

This form accompanies *Teach Me Language*. Complete instructions on its use are in Chapter 5 of *Teach Me Language*.
Copyright © 1997 SKF Books.

Letter Template

Date: ----------------------------------

Greeting: --

Body: --

Closing: --

Name: --

Letter Template This template introduces the child to letter writing. Letters can be quite structured which makes them fairly easy to master.

This form accompanies *Teach Me Language*. Complete instructions on its use are in Chapter 5 of *Teach Me Language*.
Copyright © 1997 SKF Books.

What I Did Today: (What Did You Do Today?)

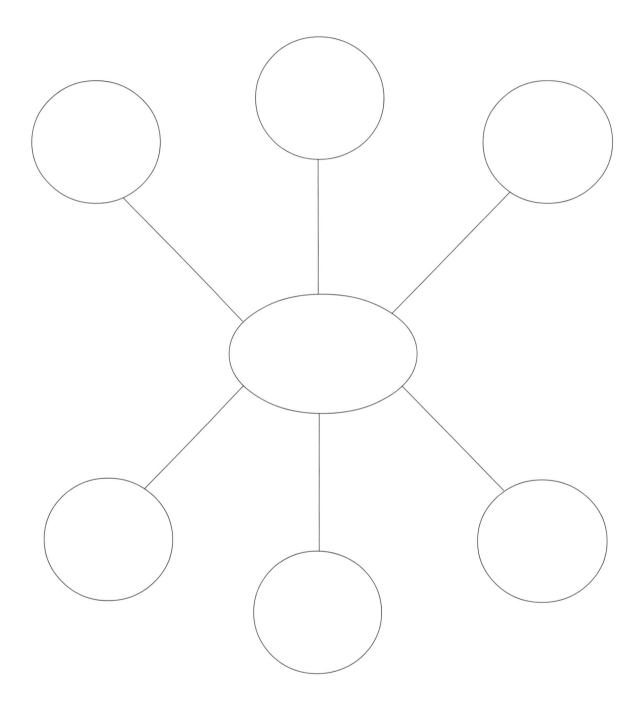

What I Did Today This form is to be used to help the child recall his/her day. Once the child remembers something, then it is written in one of the balloons. When all the spaces are full, the child uses this sheet to describe his/her day in full sentences. Then the sheet should be removed, and the child should recall that day orally (without the visual prompt). When the child can easily recall his/her day using the sheet, the sheet should not be used at all, and the child should be required to recall his day independently and orally. The eventual elimination of the sheet is very important.

This form accompanies *Teach Me Language*. Complete instructions on its use are in Chapter 5 of *Teach Me Language*. Copyright © 1997 SKF Books.

Daily Routine Sheet (Recall of Day)

What I Did Today...

Recall of Day This sheet is a written record of the child's recall of his/her day. The therapist or parent must write the child's recall, "word for word", to be able to accurately gauge progress in recall from week to week. Note that this is NOT a sheet that the child works with directly.

This form accompanies *Teach Me Language*. Complete instructions on its use are in Chapter 5 of *Teach Me Language*. Copyright © 1997 SKF Books.

6 Academics/Language Based Concepts

Forms

- Simple Categorization: Nouns
- Simple Categorization: Verbs
- Simple Categorization: Naming Items
- Familiar Words: Identifying the Group & Function
- Object Functions: Fill-Ins

- Brainstorming
- Categorization
- Pre-Reading Comprehension: Who? and What did (or do)?
- Pre-Reading Comprehension: Who? and What did (or do)?
- Important Story Events
- Story Sequence
- Story Report
- Story Summary
- Summarized Independently
- Reading Comprehension Record
- Identifying the Kind of Text Read
- Event or Details?
- Math Word Problems
- New Vocabulary
- Orally Defining Words (Objects)
- Orally Defining Words (People)
- Orally Defining Words (Verbs)
- Vocabulary and Synonyms - Easy
- Using New Vocabulary: Stories
- Applying New Vocabulary
- New Vocabulary for the Week
- New Vocabulary To Be Reinforced
- Ordering Information
- Sequencing and Ordering
- Comparing Numbers
- Understanding Place Value
- Using Comparatives - Sheet 1
- Using Comparatives - Sheet 2
- Monthly Calendar Fill-In
- Using The Correct Verb Tense

- What Happens?
- AM or PM Time
- Sequencing Time
- Comparing Time
- Time Equivalents
- Time Questions
- When Phrases
- Comparing Money - Sheet 1
- Comparing Money - Sheet 2
- Sequencing and Ordering
- Do I Have Enough Money? - Sheet 1
- Using Comparatives - Sheet 2
- Buying Things & Working with Money
- Money Questions (Auditory)
- Agents and Their Actions
- Verbal Analogies

Forms in this chapter accompany Teach Me Language. Complete instructions on their use are in Chapter 6 of Teach Me Language.
Copyright © 1997 SKF Books.

Academics/Language Based Concepts • 98

Simple Categorization: Nouns

Name 4 items in each group.

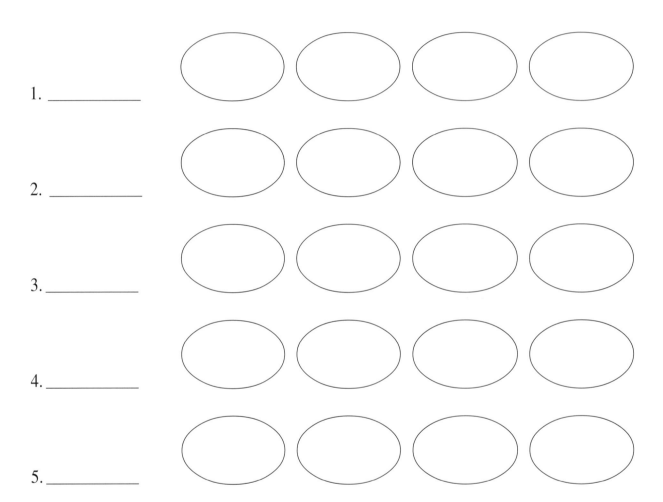

1. _____

2. _____

3. _____

4. _____

5. _____

Simple Categorization: Nouns This activity is designed to teach the child simple noun categorization. When the child can complete this exercise with ease, the next drill should be introduced. The therapist should use this drill to probe for the level of the child. If the child cannot complete this drill, then s/he should be introduced to the concepts of categories using icons, cards or 3-dimensional materials (these precursor drills must precede use of the exercises in this book).

This form accompanies *Teach Me Language*. Complete instructions on its use are in Chapter 6 of *Teach Me Language*.
Copyright © 1997 SKF Books.

Academics/Language Based Concepts • 99

Simple Categorization: Verbs

Name 4 things you can ....

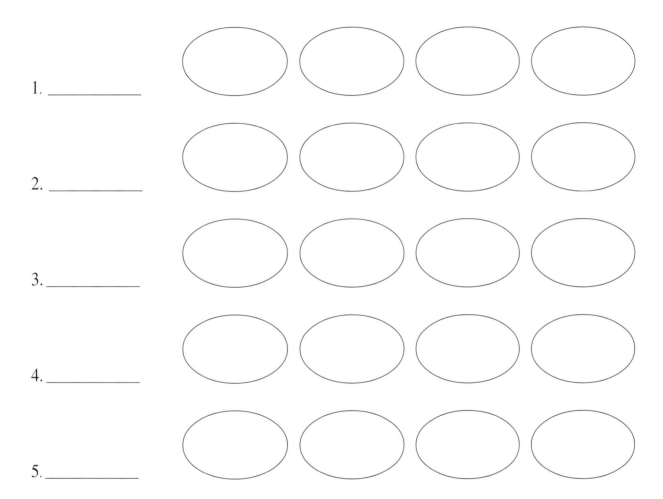

1. _____

2. _____

3. _____

4. _____

5. _____

Simple Categorization: Verbs This activity is designed to teach the child simple verb categorization. If the child can do this drill easily, the next exercise should be introduced. If the child does not understand the concept of category, then s/he needs to be introduced to categories using icons, cards or 3-dimensional materials before being introduced to the exercises in this book.

This form accompanies *Teach Me Language*. Complete instructions on its use are in Chapter 6 of *Teach Me Language*.
Copyright © 1997 SKF Books.

Academics/Language Based Concepts • 100

Simple Categorization: Naming Items

Write down three items that belong in each group.

_____   _____   _____

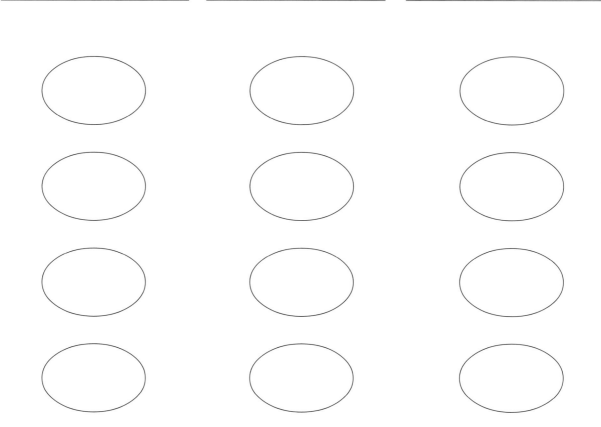

Simple Categorization: Naming Items This activity is a variation on the noun and verb categorization exercises. The focus in this drill is on the child's ability to name items that are in a category. The child should be able to complete the noun and verb categorization before being introduced to the Naming Items categorization exercise.

This form accompanies *Teach Me Language*. Complete instructions on its use are in Chapter 6 of *Teach Me Language*. Copyright © 1997 SKF Books.

Familiar Words: Identifying the Group & Function

Object   Group   Function

1._____

2._____

3._____

4._____

5._____

Familiar Words: Identifying the Group & Function This exercise is designed to teach the child the relationship between the object, the category (group) it is part of, and what it does (its function). This exercise should be introduced once the child has internalized several noun and verb categories.

This form accompanies *Teach Me Language*. Complete instructions on its use are in Chapter 6 of *Teach Me Language*. Copyright © 1997 SKF Books.

Academics/Language Based Concepts • 102

Object Functions: Fill-Ins

Complete Each Sentence.

1. _____

2. _____

3. _____

4. _____

5. _____

Object Functions: Fill-Ins This exercise is designed to teach the child the relationship between the verb (action word) and the noun. This activity requires the child to find a verb which goes with the object. If the child can write, s/he can complete the sheet independently once s/he understands the structure of the drill.

This form accompanies *Teach Me Language*. Complete instructions on its use are in Chapter 6 of *Teach Me Language*.
Copyright © 1997 SKF Books.

Academics/Language Based Concepts • 103

Categorization

Things that are (or things I do at):

_____

1. _____

2. _____

3. _____

4. _____

5. _____

Categorization This exercise teaches the child to categorize activities that occur during a period of time. The child should be able to complete the noun and verb sheets with ease before this sheet is introduced. It is important that the child retell the therapist about the topic in complete sentences, first using the sheet as a visual prompt, and then without the sheet.

This form accompanies *Teach Me Language*. Complete instructions on its use are in Chapter 6 of *Teach Me Language*.
Copyright © 1997 SKF Books.

Brainstorming

Topic: _____

○ _____   ○ _____

○ _____   ○ _____

○ _____   ○ _____

○ _____   ○ _____

○ _____   ○ _____

○ _____   ○ _____

Brainstorming This exercise teaches the child to generate ideas without being constrained by the difficulty of putting the ideas into a sentence. Once the ideas have been generated, then the child can use the key words to talk about the subject in full sentences.

This form accompanies *Teach Me Language*. Complete instructions on its use are in Chapter 6 of *Teach Me Language*. Copyright © 1997 SKF Books.

Pre-Reading Comprehension:
Who? and What did (or do)?

Circle the word(s) that answers the question.

1. _____   _____
                               _____

2. _____   _____
                               _____

3. _____   _____
                               _____

4. _____   _____
                               _____

Pre-Reading Comprehension: Who? and What did (or do)? The child should read the sentence and then answer the question by circling the correct word in the sentence. This exercise should be introduced using only "Who" questions. Once the child can complete the sheet easily answering the "Who" questions without help, the same sheet should be used asking only "What Did _____ do?" questions. Once the child can answer these questions without prompts, then the "Who" and the "What Did" questions should be mixed (as is shown on the following page).

This form accompanies *Teach Me Language*. Complete instructions on its use are in Chapter 6 of *Teach Me Language*.
Copyright © 1997 SKF Books.

Pre-Reading Comprehension:
Who? and What did (or do)?

Circle the word(s) that answers the Who question and underline the word that answers the What question. Then connect the answers to the questions with a line.

1. _____   _____
                              _____

2. _____   _____
                              _____

3. _____   _____
                              _____

4. _____   _____
                              _____

Pre-Reading Comprehension: Who? and What did (or do)? The child should read the sentence and then answer the question by circling the word in the sentence that answers the "Who" question. Next, the child should underline the word in the sentence that answers the "Did What?" question. Then, the child can draw a line connecting the noun with WHO, or the verb with the WHAT. This level of the exercise combines both "Who" and "What Did" questions in a mixed order. The therapist should keep producing new sheets in the same format (mixed questions, different persons - pronouns, noun, and proper nouns) until the child can easily complete the sheet him/herself. Once the child can complete the sheet without the therapist's prompts, it is time to start higher level reading comprehension activities (which follow).

This form accompanies *Teach Me Language*. Complete instructions on its use are in Chapter 6 of *Teach Me Language*.
Copyright © 1997 SKF Books.

Important Story Events

Title: _____	
Characters (Who)	Sequence of Events (What Happens)

Important Story Events This is the first of 4 sheets that can be used when teaching reading comprehension. This first sheet has the child name all the characters and tell what happened. The therapist should have the child stop reading every few lines to fill in this sheet. *Note: The example used in this sheet is quite high level. The story read was taken from the 5th book of 10 in level 3 of Reading Milestones. Typically, the child should start with a much lower level story.*

This form accompanies *Teach Me Language*. Complete instructions on its use are in Chapter 6 of *Teach Me Language*. Copyright © 1997 SKF Books.

Story Sequence

Title: _____

Mixed Up Order	Right Order
_____	_____
_____	_____
_____	_____
_____	_____
_____	_____

What happened first?_____
_____

What happened last? _____
_____

Story Sequence This is the second of 4 sheets that should be used when teaching reading comprehension. The second sheet requires the child take all the major events in the story and put them in the correct order. This is a particularly important skill for the child to master since ability to sequence is inextricably linked to story comprehension. It is important that the therapist write up the mixed order of story events before beginning the entire comprehension exercise with the child.

This form accompanies *Teach Me Language*. Complete instructions on its use are in Chapter 6 of *Teach Me Language*.
Copyright © 1997 SKF Books.

Story Report

Date:

Title of the book: _____

Author: _____

My prediction: I think the book is about _____

_____

It was about:

    WHO? _____

    WHERE? _____

    WHAT HAPPENED? _____

FIRST _____

THEN _____

LAST _____

WHAT I LIKED ABOUT THE BOOK: I liked the book because _____

_____

Story Report This is the third of 4 sheets that should be used when teaching reading comprehension. The third sheet requires the child to report on the story by asking him/her to answer assorted important questions about the story such as Who, Where, and What Happened. The structure created by this form helps clarify the story to the child. This sheet will help the child throughout his/her schooling since the child will be asked to read and report on books in several grades.

This form accompanies *Teach Me Language*. Complete instructions on its use are in Chapter 6 of *Teach Me Language*.
Copyright © 1997 SKF Books.

Story Summary

The story _____ takes

place _____. The main

character _____ who _____

_____.

In this story _____

_____

_____

At the end, _____

_____

_____

Story Summary This is the fourth sheet in the series that can be used when teaching reading comprehension. This form has the child briefly summarize the story in a structured way. This last sheet tells the therapist how much of the story was understood. If the child is not able to comprehend the story (as evidenced by this last sheet), then the next story chosen should be much shorter and at a lower level using the same four sheet system.

This form accompanies *Teach Me Language*. Complete instructions on its use are in Chapter 6 of *Teach Me Language*.
Copyright © 1997 SKF Books.

Summarizing Independently

Read the story sequence. Tell what the story is about.

The story is about ─────────────────────────────────────

        ─────────────────────────────────────

        ─────────────────────────────────────

        ─────────────────────────────────────

        ─────────────────────────────────────

        ─────────────────────────────────────

Summarizing Independently When the child is able to complete the 3 or 4 forms that precede the Story Summary sheet, then s/he should be given the opportunity to independently complete this form. This is a very advanced skill since it works on an important deficit - sequencing - which is very difficult for so many language delayed children. Once the child completes this form, he should then be required to verbally summarize the story without the form.

This form accompanies *Teach Me Language*. Complete instructions on its use are in Chapter 6 of *Teach Me Language*.
Copyright © 1997 SKF Books.

Reading Comprehension Record

Story: _____   Date started: _____
    Book: _____
    ☐ Predict
    ☐ Read
    ☐ Important Story Events Notes   ☐ Reading Notes
    ☐ Work sheets
    ☐ Comparison
    ☐ Mixed Order - Sequencing
    ☐ Story Comprehension Form   ☐ Outline
    ☐ P/S Comprehension Form   ☐ Descriptive Paragraph
    ☐ Story Summary

    Notes: _____   Date Completed: _____

Story: _____   Date started: _____
    Book: _____
    ☐ Predict
    ☐ Read
    ☐ Important Story Events Notes   ☐ Reading Notes
    ☐ Work sheets
    ☐ Comparison
    ☐ Mixed Order - Sequencing
    ☐ Story Comprehension Form   ☐ Outline
    ☐ P/S Comprehension Form   ☐ Descriptive Paragraph
    ☐ Story Summary

    Notes: _____   Date Completed: _____

Story: _____   Date started: _____
    Book: _____
    ☐ Predict
    ☐ Read
    ☐ Important Story Events Notes   ☐ Reading Notes
    ☐ Work sheets
    ☐ Comparison
    ☐ Mixed Order - Sequencing
    ☐ Story Comprehension Form   ☐ Outline
    ☐ P/S Comprehension Form   ☐ Descriptive Paragraph
    ☐ Story Summary

    Notes: _____   Date Completed: _____

Reading Comprehension Record This sheet is designed to keep track of the stories and exercises completed with each story. If one person is in charge of the reading comprehension, this record is not critical; however, if a number of people are working with the child, it is important to keep a record of the stories completed so that 1) there is no duplication and 2) the child does all the exercises appropriate for his/her level (this will vary from child to child).

This form accompanies *Teach Me Language*. Complete instructions on its use are in Chapter 6 of *Teach Me Language*.
Copyright © 1997 SKF Books.

Identifying the Kind of Text Read

Date: _____

Look at each title. Tell whether the title tells you if what is read will be a STORY, a DESCRIPTIVE/FACTUAL paragraph, a COMPARATIVE paragraph or a "HOW TO" paragraph.

Title	Type of Paragraph(s)/Text

Give an example of a title for a story, descriptive/factual paragraph, comparative paragraph, or "how to" paragraph:

_____

_____

Identifying the Kind of Text Read This sheet is designed to teach the child to identify the type of text that s/he is reading. This is an important skill because it will determine how the child goes about understanding the text. For example, if the text is a story, then sequence is important; whereas, if the text is factual, there is often no real sequence to understand.

This form accompanies *Teach Me Language*. Complete instructions on its use are in Chapter 6 of *Teach Me Language*.
Copyright © 1997 SKF Books.

Event or Detail?

Read each sentence from a story. Tell whether it is an event of the story or a detail.
Then recall one more event and one more detail from the story.

Story: _____   Event or Detail?

_____   _____

_____   _____

_____   _____

Event in: _____   _____

_____

Detail in: _____   _____

_____

Event or Detail? This exercise is designed to teach the child to identify whether the sentence describes an event or a detail in the story. This is an important skill because if the child concentrates on each sentence of the story equally, it will be very hard to comprehend the story. **The child needs to be told and remember that an action is always an event, and a description is always a detail.** The therapist should ask: Why is this an event? (because it happened). Why is this a detail? (because it is a description).

This form accompanies *Teach Me Language*. Complete instructions on its use are in Chapter 6 of *Teach Me Language*.
Copyright © 1997 SKF Books.

Math Word Problems

Number Equation   Key Word(s)

_____   _____

Word Problem: _____

_____

_____

Number Equation   Key Word(s)

_____   _____

Word Problem: _____

_____

_____

Math Word Problems   The Math Problem exercise is designed to teach reading comprehension by pairing words to symbols. Once the child has learned the key words for addition, then the key words for subtraction can be taught. Math word problems are a particular challenge for children with language disorders even if they are good at math. This exercise makes math problems easier to understand and complete.

This form accompanies *Teach Me Language*. Complete instructions on its use are in Chapter 6 of *Teach Me Language*.
Copyright © 1997 SKF Books.

New Vocabulary

_____   _____
(New word)

                                    _____
                                    (Definition of new word)

Descriptions e.g. things you can do with a _____; where you see a _____; who has a _____, what goes in a _____, etc...

New word used in sentences:

_____

_____

_____

New Vocabulary This exercise teaches new noun vocabulary and works on the concept that words can be defined. First, the child should be instructed to define the word. Then, the therapist should choose two descriptions and have the child give suggestions as to the function of the object or give a description of the object. It is important to introduce words the child already knows since the skill to be learned is defining words or understanding that words have definitions. Later, words that the child does not know can be introduced with the use of this sheet and a child's dictionary.

This form accompanies *Teach Me Language*. Complete instructions on its use are in Chapter 6 of *Teach Me Language*.
Copyright © 1997 SKF Books.

Academics/Language Based Concepts • 117

Orally Defining Words (Objects)

Title: _____

Description   Group   Use

Tell something about it;   What do you do with it?
                                                 use 1 or 2 adjectives

_____   _____   _____

_____   _____   _____

Definition: A _____ is a _____ that

_____

Sentences

Home: _____

School: _____

Community: _____

Orally Defining Words (Objects) This vocabulary exercise gives the child the opportunity to learn to define objects by what they do or by which group they belong to. Then, the sheet instructs the child to use the word in sentences relating to a variety of settings. This sheet should not be introduced to the child until the child has finished the Community script in Chapter 3. Once the child has completed the form, s/he should define the word, first using the form as a visual cue, and then, without the form.

This form accompanies *Teach Me Language*. Complete instructions on its use are in Chapter 6 of *Teach Me Language*.
Copyright © 1997 SKF Books.

Orally Defining Words (People)

Title: _____

Description   Group   Is/Has/Does

Use male or female

_____   _____   _____

_____

Definition: A _____ is a _____ that

_____

Sentences

Home: _____

School: _____

Community: _____

Orally Defining Words (People) This vocabulary exercise gives the child the opportunity to learn to define people by what they are and by which group they belong to. Then, the sheet instructs the child to use the word in a sentence as it relates to a variety of settings. This sheet should not be introduced to the child until the child has finished the Community script in Chapter 3. The child should orally define the word, first using the sheet and then, without the sheet.

This form accompanies *Teach Me Language*. Complete instructions on its use are in Chapter 6 of *Teach Me Language*.
Copyright © 1997 SKF Books.

Orally Defining Words (Verbs)

Title: _____

Verb/Action   Done with   Purpose

                        body part or object   lets you ...

_____   _____   _____

_____

Definition: _____ is something you do with

_____ to _____

Home: _____

School: _____

Community: _____

Orally Defining Words (Verbs) This vocabulary exercise gives the child the opportunity to learn to define verbs by what they are for (their purpose) and which body part one does them with. Then the sheet has the child use the word in sentences relating to a variety of settings. This sheet should not be introduced to the child until the child has finished the Community script in Chapter 3. The child should orally define the word, first using the sheet and then, without the sheet.

This form accompanies *Teach Me Language*. Complete instructions on its use are in Chapter 6 of *Teach Me Language*.
Copyright © 1997 SKF Books.

Vocabulary and Synonyms - Easy

Write down a synonym - a word that means the same thing as the word listed. Then use the new word in a sentence.

New Word - Synonym   Sentence

_____   _____

_____   _____

_____   _____

_____   _____

_____   _____

_____   _____

Vocabulary and Synonyms - Easy This new vocabulary exercise requires the child to use all the words s/he has learned through the new vocabulary sheets by finding a word that means the same thing and then using the word in a sentence. This should be done with the words that have been introduced through the new vocabulary sheets. This should NOT be done with any words that have not been introduced in this way since it will be very difficult for the child to come up with synonyms by him/herself without knowing the definition of a word.

This form accompanies *Teach Me Language*. Complete instructions on its use are in Chapter 6 of *Teach Me Language*. Copyright © 1997 SKF Books.

Academics/Language Based Concepts • 121

Using New Vocabulary: Stories

Use these words in a short story: _____

Title: _____

Prompts:

| Who | Did What | When | Why |

_____

_____

_____

_____

_____

Using New Vocabulary: Stories This vocabulary exercise gives the child the opportunity to use the words s/he has learned in a story. Through this exercise, the child learns that those words found in a story are relevant and can be used in other stories. In addition, this exercise strengthens the child's comprehension of the word so that when the child sees the word in a new story, s/he will understand it.

This form accompanies *Teach Me Language*. Complete instructions on its use are in Chapter 6 of *Teach Me Language*.
Copyright © 1997 SKF Books.

Academics/Language Based Concepts • 122

Applying New Vocabulary

Tell how you would apply or use each word at home, at school, or out in the community.

Word	Home	School	Community
_____			
_____			
_____			

Applying New Vocabulary The Applying New Vocabulary exercise requires the child to use all the words s/he has learned through the new vocabulary sheets in three different settings. This should be done with all applicable words that have been introduced through the new vocabulary exercises.

This form accompanies *Teach Me Language*. Complete instructions on its use are in Chapter 6 of *Teach Me Language*. Copyright © 1997 SKF Books.

New Vocabulary for the Week

1. Define the word.
2. Write down what kind of word it is.
3. Write down where or how you would use the word.

Word	Definition	Kind of Word	Where/ How Might Use/Apply the Word
_____			
_____			
_____			

New Vocabulary for the Week This exercise has the child provide a synonym for the weekly words (thereby defining the word), identify the kind of word it is (its function) and apply the word in any way the child is able. This is a much more difficult vocabulary exercise than the previous exercises since it concentrates on the skills used in several drills. When the child can easily complete the easier vocabulary drills, this drill should be introduced and done with <u>all</u> new vocabulary words introduced to the child. This exercise should NOT be done with any words that have not been introduced through the other exercises.

This form accompanies *Teach Me Language*. Complete instructions on its use are in Chapter 6 of *Teach Me Language*.
Copyright © 1997 SKF Books.

New Vocabulary To Be Reinforced

New Word - Definition or Word Paired With

New Word - Definition or Word Paired With

New Vocabulary To Be Reinforced This vocabulary sheet is provided as a therapy record to keep track of all the vocabulary words that have been recently introduced. This is not a form the child should work with.

This form accompanies *Teach Me Language*. Complete instructions on its use are in Chapter 6 of *Teach Me Language*. Copyright © 1997 SKF Books.

Academics/Language Based Concepts • 125

Ordering Information

Follow each direction. Put the items in order. Use a 1 (first), 2 (second), 3 (third) order.

1. Order these _____ from _____ to _____   _____

   _____

   _____

2. Order these _____ from _____ to _____   _____

   _____

   _____

3. Order these _____ from _____ to _____   _____

   _____

   _____

Ordering Information This exercise has the child order information given in a specified sequence. In this example, the therapist gives all the information out of order and the child is required to number the information according to the instructions.

This form accompanies *Teach Me Language*. Complete instructions on its use are in Chapter 6 of *Teach Me Language*.
Copyright © 1997 SKF Books.

Academics/Language Based Concepts • 126

Sequencing and Ordering

Read each direction and order the _____ by writing 1, 2, 3, and 4 in the correct boxes.

Sequencing and Ordering This exercise, like the one before it, has the child order the information given in a specified sequence. In this example, the therapist concentrates on the concept of relative age. This exercise can also be used with numbers.

This form accompanies *Teach Me Language*. Complete instructions on its use are in Chapter 6 of *Teach Me Language*.
Copyright © 1997 SKF Books.

Comparing Numbers

Look at each number. Count the number of digits in each number. Circle the number that is bigger or smaller, higher or lower.

_____   _____   _____   _____

_____   _____   _____   _____

_____   _____   _____   _____

_____   _____   _____   _____

_____   _____   _____   _____

Write a number that is _____ than _____. _____

Write a number that is _____ than _____. _____

Write a number that is _____ than _____. _____

Write a number that is _____ than _____. _____

Write a number that is _____ than _____. _____

Write a number that is _____ than _____. _____

Comparing Numbers This exercise provides a way to practice skills gained in the number sequencing and ordering drills. The Comparing Numbers exercise is also another way to strengthen new knowledge the child has gained about place value and sequencing (which follows).

This form accompanies *Teach Me Language*. Complete instructions on its use are in Chapter 6 of *Teach Me Language*. Copyright © 1997 SKF Books.

Understanding Place Value

Look at each number. Tell how many digits it has. Then tell what each digit means.

Number	How many digits	What each digit means

Number   How many digits   What each digit means

_____ _____

                                                                  _____ one thousands

                                                                  _____ one hundreds

                                                                  _____ tens

                                                                  _____ ones

_____ _____

                                                                  _____ one thousands

                                                                  _____ one hundreds

                                                                  _____ tens

                                                                  _____ ones

Understanding Place Value The Understanding Place Value exercise reinforces what has been learned in the Place Value script. The goal is for the child to understand what the number means to prevent him/her from falling behind in math due to difficulty in grasping language based math concepts.

This form accompanies *Teach Me Language*. Complete instructions on its use are in Chapter 6 of *Teach Me Language*. Copyright © 1997 SKF Books.

Academics/Language Based Concepts • 129

Using Comparatives - Sheet 1

Look at the comparative adjectives on the line. Use one of the comparative words to make a sentence about the two word pairs.

Comparatives: _____

_____

_____   _____

_____   _____

_____   _____

_____

_____

_____

_____

Using Comparatives - Sheet 1 This exercise has the child compare relative size by using material that the child is familiar with, in this case animal size. When preparing this sheet, the therapist should draw lines from one adjective to another, making sure that there are obvious differences in what is being compared.

This form accompanies *Teach Me Language*. Complete instructions on its use are in Chapter 6 of *Teach Me Language*.
Copyright © 1997 SKF Books.

Academics/Language Based Concepts ● 130

Using Comparatives - Sheet 2

Put the _____, _____ things under the correct box.

[ ]   [ ]   [ ]

_____

Which is _____

Which is _____

Is the _____ than the _____

Is the _____ than the _____

Think of something that is _____

Think of something that is _____

Put the 3 things in order from _____

_____

_____

_____

Using Comparatives - Sheet 2 This exercise has the child compare relative size using three objects. This is a much more difficult exercise than the Using Comparatives - Sheet 1 because the child must 1) order three objects, and 2) generate original ideas about the relationship of the objects to other items. The therapist writes the questions and the child answers orally.

This form accompanies *Teach Me Language*. Complete instructions on its use are in Chapter 6 of *Teach Me Language*.
Copyright © 1997 SKF Books.

Academics/Language Based Concepts • 131

Monthly Calendar Fill-In

Read each sentence. Fill in the correct answer.

There are _____ days in _____.

The first day of _____ is on a _____day.

The last day of _____ is on a _____day.

The _____ of _____ is on a _____day.

The _____ of _____ is on a _____day.

There are _____ _____days in _____.

There are _____ _____days in _____.

_____ is the month before _____.

_____ is the month after _____.

Monthly Calendar Fill-In At the beginning of every month, the child should complete this sheet using a calendar to refer to. This will help maintain the calendar skills learned from the calendar script and calendar drills. Eventually, the child should be able to know, without looking at a calendar, the month before and the month after the current month. Other than that the child SHOULD NOT be encouraged to memorize mundane calendar facts (e.g. how many Mondays there are in August).

This form accompanies *Teach Me Language*. Complete instructions on its use are in Chapter 6 of *Teach Me Language*.
Copyright © 1997 SKF Books.

# Using The Correct Verb Tense

Read each sentence. Circle the correct verb tense.

_____

_____

_____

_____

Complete each sentence (let the child use his personal calendar initially).

_____

_____

Using The Correct Verb Tense This exercise works on the child's verb tenses. The sheet should be customized to the child in order for the verb tenses to have meaning. If the child is supposed to conjugate a verb with "Yesterday", the therapist must use a verb that reflects what the child did yesterday. The more the therapist can relate the child's experience with the language being taught, the more sense that concept will make to the child.

Note: The therapist should set up the sheet to reflect the concepts that the child is working on at the moment.

This form accompanies *Teach Me Language*. Complete instructions on its use are in Chapter 6 of *Teach Me Language*.
Copyright © 1997 SKF Books.

Academics/Language Based Concepts • 133

What Happens?

Look at each period of time and answer the question.

What _____?   Event

_____   _____

_____   _____

_____   _____

_____   _____

When _____?   _____
When _____?   _____

What Happens? This exercise has the child match a period of time with an activity that the child does at that time. Each sheet needs to be customized to the specific child. For example, if the child goes to gymnastics on Saturday morning, the therapist should use Saturday morning as one of the periods of time to describe the event. The more meaningful the activities and the more varied the times, the greater likelihood that the child will understand this concept.

This form accompanies *Teach Me Language*. Complete instructions on its use are in Chapter 6 of *Teach Me Language*.
Copyright © 1997 SKF Books.

AM Or PM Time

Look at each event or thing that happens.
Tell whether the event happens in the A.M. or P.M.

Event   A.M. or P.M.?

_____   _____

_____   _____

_____   _____

_____   _____

_____   _____

What is something you might do during A.M. hours?

_____

What is something you might do during P.M. hours?

_____

AM Or PM Time This exercise has the child match an activity to the A.M. or P.M. This is a much harder exercise than the previous one because the concept of A.M. and P.M. is abstract. Before this exercise is introduced, the child must be shown on a blackboard or piece of paper that A.M. refers to all time from 12:00 in the early morning to 11:59 in the late morning, and that P.M. refers to all time from 12:00 noon (lunchtime) to 11:59 at night. Although this is a Sequencing A Day exercise, it should not be introduced until the child is learning "Time".

This form accompanies *Teach Me Language*. Complete instructions on its use are in Chapter 6 of *Teach Me Language*.
Copyright © 1997 SKF Books.

Sequencing Time

Put the time amounts in order from: _____

_____   _____ _____ _____

_____   _____ _____ _____

_____   _____ _____ _____

_____   _____ _____ _____

Sequencing Time In this exercise, the child sequences time according to the instructions at the top of the sheet which are customized by the therapist based on the Teaching Time Hierarchy. The example uses "shorter to longer" time amounts. The child should also sequence "longer to shorter", "less time" to "more time", and "more time" to "less time".

This form accompanies *Teach Me Language*. Complete instructions on its use are in Chapter 6 of *Teach Me Language*.
Copyright © 1997 SKF Books.

Comparing Time

Look at each amount of time.
Circle the amount that:

_____   _____   _____   _____

_____   _____   _____   _____

_____   _____   _____   _____

_____   _____   _____   _____

Comparing Time In this exercise the child compares time by its relative length. This should be relatively easy for the child if s/he has mastered time using the time cards. If this drill is difficult, the therapist should return to the cards for a refresher session.

This form accompanies *Teach Me Language*. Complete instructions on its use are in Chapter 6 of *Teach Me Language*.
Copyright © 1997 SKF Books.

Time Equivalents

Look at each amount of time.
Circle the amount or amounts of time that are the same.

_____   _____   _____   _____   _____

_____   _____   _____   _____   _____

_____   _____   _____   _____   _____

_____   _____   _____   _____   _____

Time Equivalents In this exercise the child identifies the amount of time that is equivalent to the amount of time on the left-hand side of the page. This drill should be relatively easy for the child if s/he has learned time from the cards. If the child has difficulty completing this drill, the therapist should return to the cards until the child has mastered time using the time cards.

This form accompanies *Teach Me Language*. Complete instructions on its use are in Chapter 6 of *Teach Me Language*.
Copyright © 1997 SKF Books.

Time Questions

Which takes longer, brushing your teeth or taking a bath? _____

Which takes less time, typing your shoes or watching the Jungle Book? _____

Which takes longer, baking a cake or eating a bowl or cereal? _____

Which takes less time, doing your homework, or brushing your hair? _____

Which is the most amount of time - 24 hours or 2 days? _____

How many days are in a week? _____

How many hours in a day? _____

How many seconds in a minute? _____

How many months in a year? _____

How many days in a month? _____

What happens at school at 10 o'clock? _____

What happens at around 8:30? _____

What time is morning recess? _____

What time does school start? _____

When is lunch? _____

What do you do at about 10:30? _____

Time Questions This exercise has the child think about the concept of time by comparing amounts of time. The exercise also helps maintain what the child has learned about time from the preceding exercises. These questions are asked orally to the child. The question sheet should be customized to the specific child, where appropriate.

This form accompanies *Teach Me Language*. Complete instructions on its use are in Chapter 6 of *Teach Me Language*. Copyright © 1997 SKF Books.

When Phrases

Write down 3 things that you do:

_____   _____

1. _____   1. _____

2. _____   2. _____

3. _____   3. _____

When Phrases This exercise has the child list activities that s/he does at certain times of the day. Other times of the day that can be used in the exercise are: at breakfast, at recess, at lunch, at dinner, in the evening, after school, on Saturday (any day of the week), before school, before bedtime, during recess, etc.

This form accompanies *Teach Me Language*. Complete instructions on its use are in Chapter 6 of *Teach Me Language*.
Copyright © 1997 SKF Books.

Comparing Money - Sheet 1

Look at each amount of money.
Circle the amount that:

_____   _____   _____   _____

_____   _____   _____   _____

_____   _____   _____   _____

_____   _____   _____   _____

Comparing Money - Sheet 1 The money comparison exercise gives the child practice at looking at relative amounts and discerning their relative value. It is important that the child have this concept firmly internalized before s/he can use money independently.

This form accompanies *Teach Me Language*. Complete instructions on its use are in Chapter 6 of *Teach Me Language*. Copyright © 1997 SKF Books.

Academics/Language Based Concepts • 141

Comparing Money - Sheet 2

Look at each amount of money.
Circle the amount that:

Comparing Money - Sheet 2 This second money comparison exercise is much harder than the first because the amounts are larger and more complex. It is important for the child to be able to do this drill very easily before the concepts of "enough money" and "change back" are introduced.

This form accompanies *Teach Me Language*. Complete instructions on its use are in Chapter 6 of *Teach Me Language*.
Copyright © 1997 SKF Books.

Academics/Language Based Concepts • 142

Sequencing And Ordering

Read each direction and order the _____ by writing 1, 2, 3, and 4 in the correct boxes.

Sequencing And Ordering This exercise has the child order numbers or money in a particular sequence. In this example, the therapist concentrates on the concept of relative prices.

This form accompanies *Teach Me Language*. Complete instructions on its use are in Chapter 6 of *Teach Me Language*. Copyright © 1997 SKF Books.

… 143

Do I Have Enough Money? - Sheet 1

When you want to buy something, you have to figure out if you have enough money to buy it.

Item   Cost   Money I have

_____   _____   _____

                                                _____

                                                _____

Total Money I have ⟶ ☐

(circle one)

Do I have enough money to buy _____ ?   Yes/No
                                (item)

Which do I have? (circle one)

- Less Than Enough

- More Than Enough

- Just Enough
  (the same amount as the cost)

> If I have **less than enough money**, how much **more money** do I need?
>
> Cost of _____   ☐
>
> How much money do I have?   ☐
>
> How much more money do I need? ☐

Do I Have Enough Money? - Sheet 1 This exercise is designed to give the child the tools s/he needs to grasp the concept of "enough money". The therapist should go through the drill several times with the child until s/he understands the concept. The next step is to play "store" with the therapist and then with a peer. Once the child can do the sheet relatively well and can pretend play "store", the s/he can be taken to a restaurant or store. The child should order something and compute the change s/he should receive. By making this realistic, the child will understand and be motivated to use this skill, especially to make sure s/he has enough money for the purchase of choice.

This form accompanies *Teach Me Language*. Complete instructions on its use are in Chapter 6 of *Teach Me Language*.
Copyright © 1997 SKF Books.

Do I Have Enough Money - Sheet 2

When you want to buy something, you have to figure out if you have enough money to buy it.

Item	Cost	Money I have
_____	_____	_____
		_____
		_____

Total Money I have ⟶ ☐

(circle one)

Do I have enough money to buy _____ ?   **Yes/No**
_(item)

Which do I have? (circle one)

- Less Than Enough
- More Than Enough
- Just Enough
  (the same amount as the cost)

If I have **less than enough money**, how much **more money** do I need?	If I have **more than enough money**, how much **change** do I get back?

Cost of _____ ☐
     (item)
How much money do I have? ☐
How much more money do I need? ☐
	How much money do I have? ☐
	Cost of _____ ☐
	     (item)
	How much change do I get back? ☐

This more difficult exercise is designed to teach the child 1) whether or not s/he has enough money, and 2) when s/he has too much money, how much change s/he should get back. The therapist should go through the drill several times with the child until s/he understands the concept of "getting change back". Once the child can do this drill easily, then s/he should start incorporating this skill into his/her daily life (every time the child goes to a store or restaurant).

This form accompanies *Teach Me Language*. Complete instructions on its use are in Chapter 6 of *Teach Me Language*.
Copyright © 1997 SKF Books.

Academics/Language Based Concepts • 145

Buying Things & Working With Money

You want to buy these things: Cost:

1. _____ $ _____
    (item)
2. _____ $ _____
    (item)
3. _____ $ _____
    (item)

What is the TOTAL COST? ⟶ $ _____

What is the largest bill you will need?   (circle one)

$1 $% $10 $20

If you have $ _____, will you have enough money to buy the items? _____
If you have $ _____, will you have enough money to buy the items? _____
If you have $ _____, will you have more or less money than you need? _____
If you have $ _____, will you have more or less money than you need? _____

If you want to give the cashier the EXACT AMOUNT OF MONEY, what would you give her?

Number of bills or coins: _____ dollars = $ _____
                          _____ quarters = $ _____
                          _____ dimes   = $ _____
                          _____ nickels = $ _____
                          _____ pennies = $ _____

Total ⟶ _____

If you gave the cashier $ _____,, how much change would you get back?

Amount you give the cashier   _____
The cost of the items (substract)   −   _____

Change you should get back ⟶ _____

Buying Things & Working With Money This exercises builds on the previous exercises. In this exercise the child learns to use money when there is more than one item being bought. Incorporated into this exercise is the concept of "enough money", "change back", and "total cost".

This form accompanies *Teach Me Language*. Complete instructions on its use are in Chapter 6 of *Teach Me Language*.
Copyright © 1997 SKF Books.

Money Questions (Auditory)

Which is worth the most, _____?

Which is worth the least, _____?

Which is the higher price, _____?

Which is the lower price, _____?

Which costs more, _____?

Which costs more, your school lunch or a candy bar?

Which costs less, a coke or a happy meal?

Money Questions (Auditory) This exercise has the child listen and then answer questions which ask about the relative worth of money. These questions should be customized to the individual child so that the questions relate to his/her life. This auditory drill should not be done with the child until the preceding written exercises on relative value of money are understood completely by the child.

This form accompanies *Teach Me Language*. Complete instructions on its use are in Chapter 6 of *Teach Me Language*.
Copyright © 1997 SKF Books.

…
Agents and Their Actions

Agent: _____ (person, place, thing)

Things _____ can do	Things _____ can't do

Questions

Why can't _____ ? _____

Why can't _____ ? _____

Why can't _____ ? _____

Agents and Their Actions This exercise teaches the child about verbs and verb agents (those who do the action). The child is to name all the different things that an agent can do and a number of things that an agent cannot do. Then the child is asked to answer why the agent cannot do the various things that the child suggests.

This form accompanies *Teach Me Language*. Complete instructions on its use are in Chapter 6 of *Teach Me Language*.
Copyright © 1997 SKF Books.

Verbal Analogies

Type: _____

_____

_____

_____

_____

My own _____ analogy:

_____

_____

Verbal Analogies This exercise teaches the concept of an analogy. This is a difficult concept that can be made easy by using extremely obvious analogies about function. Once the child understands these very easy analogies, the analogies can be made less obvious. It is important to remember, however, that most normally developing children do not have a good grasp of abstract analogies.

This form accompanies *Teach Me Language*. Complete instructions on its use are in Chapter 6 of *Teach Me Language*.
Copyright © 1997 SKF Books.

7 Therapy Schedules

Forms

- Simplified Schedule for the Child
- Independent Work Instrument
- Weekly Drill/Activity Record

Forms in this chapter accompany <u>Teach Me Language</u>. Complete instructions on their use are in Chapter 7 of <u>Teach Me Language.</u>
Copyright © 1997 SKF Books.

Therapy Schedules • 150

Simplified Schedule For The Child

1 Read about _____

2 Make an outline and talk about _____

3 Write a story _____

4 Answer questions _____

5 _____

6 Talk about what I did today

7 Practice talking and having a conversation

8 _____

9 Work by myself: do independent work

When I am done, I get to: _____

Today's Work Schedule This is a sample of a therapy schedule that the child can relate to. In this way, the child see what is on the agenda and knows that in order to receive the reward at the bottom of the page, s/he must go through the schedule. The treat at the bottom should be something the child chooses (within reason) so that the child is motivated.

This form accompanies *Teach Me Language*. Complete instructions on its use are in Chapter 7 of *Teach Me Language*.
Copyright © 1997 SKF Books.

Independent Work Instrument

Check off each square when you are done.

☐ _____

☐ _____

☐ _____

☐ _____

Let me know when you are done.

Independent Work Instrument This sheet is designed to teach the child to do his/her work independently. This is also a good check as to whether the child is becoming too dependent on the therapist to complete his/her work. The items to put on the independent work sheet are drills that the child has mastered and can do ALONE without any help. The therapist should NOT have the child work on difficult activities independently since this will create frustration rather than a sense of accomplishment.

This form accompanies *Teach Me Language*. Complete instructions on its use are in Chapter 7 of *Teach Me Language*.
Copyright © 1997 SKF Books.

Weekly Drill/Activity Record

Week of: _____

Goal Areas	How Often	S	M	T	W	TH	F	S
Reading - Stories								
Reading - Topic Based								
Language								
Critical Thinking								
Conversation								

Notes: _____
_____
_____

Therapy Schedule The weekly schedule is designed for the therapy manager to monitor how often various activities are being done.

This form accompanies *Teach Me Language*. Complete instructions on its use are in Chapter 7 of *Teach Me Language*.
Copyright © 1997 SKF Books.